A Practical Guide
to Art Therapy Groups

A Practical Guide to Art Therapy Groups

Diane Fausek, BA, ADC

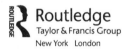

Routledge
Taylor & Francis Group
New York   London

First published 1997 by

The Haworth Press, Inc., 10 Alice Street, Binghamton, NY 13904-1580

This edition published 2014 by Routledge

Routledge
Taylor & Francis Group
711 Third Avenue
New York, NY 10017

Routledge
Taylor & Francis Group
27 Church Road, Hove
East Sussex BN3 2FA

Routledge is an imprint of the Taylor & Francis Group, an informa business

Cover design by Donna M. Brooks.

Library of Congress Cataloging-in-Publication Data

Fausek, Diane.
    A practical guide to art therapy / Diane Fausek.
        p.   cm.
    Includes index.
    ISBN 0-7890-0186-1 (alk. paper) ISBN 0-7890-0136-5 (alk. paper)
    1. Art therapy. I. Title
    RC489.A7F38 1997
    615.8'5156–dc20   96-34526
                                                                  CIP

This book is dedicated to my parents,
who taught me that laughter is always the best medicine,
and to Bill,
who makes sure I get my daily dosage.

ABOUT THE AUTHOR

Diane Fausek, BA, ADC, is Art Therapist at the Mt. Carmel Health and Rehabilitation Center in Milwaukee, Wisconsin. She holds a BA in art therapy and behavioral science and is also a certified activity director. Ms. Fausek has been practicing art therapy for over ten years. A specialist who works with geriatric, geri-psychiatric, long-term care, and rehabilitation clients, she has spoken at conferences for the Adult Daycare Association of Wisconsin and the National Therapeutic Recreation Association. She currently writes a column for *Creative Forecasting Inc.*

CONTENTS

A WORD ABOUT ADAPTATIONS

Just about any process can be adapted. It just takes some imagination and a knowledge of possible resources available. All the processes described in this book have been used with various cognitively skilled clients and many victims of one-sided paralysis due to stroke or brain injury. Routinely, I use simple sandbags with cloth covers as a third hand to keep paper from being pushed away from them while working. For more demanding processes, such as "Stringing Along," I adapted traditional embroidery hoop stands to serve as a clamp for lightweight matte frames. Many times, helpful occupational health workers and/or catalogs will have tools that can be used for art making, such as adaptive pencil holders and tray tables. When all else fails and your clients really need two hands (or more?) to be successful, plan ahead, remember to offer the valuable experience of hands-on work with clients to art students or interns from the community. This will help you and provide great stimulation and a feeling of partnership with your clients.

Good luck!
Diane

Chapter 1

Finding the Key

Art therapy is a tool that combines the creative processes of the individual, therapeutic interventions, and traditional and non-traditional art media. Art therapy has been proven successful in helping participants to learn, reach out, and to grow. It opens the door to communication between therapist and client, child and parent, individual and individual, and most important, allows us to look deep within ourselves and see truths we sometimes overlook.

Art therapy is utilized in many settings and, with adaptations, can be seen as a tool used with everyone. I have been working in long-term care for many years and know that sometimes creating original, successful, and therapeutic treatment plans can be difficult when you are working with clients with challenges of the physical, cognitive, and psychological nature. It has been with this in mind that this book originated.

Within these pages, you will find treatment plans originally used in long-term care settings, specifically with clients affected by Alzheimer's disease, complications from stroke, geri-psych, and developmentally disabled. Each one can be adapted to fit the setting you need. Each plan has a brief description of the process, followed by a materials list and sequential information on the actual implementation of the process. All processes are noted to describe the target population and requirements. All the basics are there; you just add your therapeutic skills and caring nature to provide a beneficial experience.

Using art in therapy is not without risks however, and this book is not meant to replace therapeutic training. The processes in this book have been created and implemented successfully with the long-term care clients with whom I work. I have learned that truly knowing your clients is inspiration enough to develop treatment plans to target their issues of loss, grief, lack of control, frustration, hopelessness, and life review. It is in our best interests to look at who we are, what motivates us, and how we interact with others so that we can live more successfully and feel more content with the choices we make.

I have been fortunate enough to have developed a cohesive group of clients who are supportive of each other and comfortable with expressing their issues. I am always amazed, when I am thrust into a client role by a sadistic intern, at how difficult it is to open up, and yet how easily my clients will do it. This, I know, is unusual.

HOW TO DEAL WITH THE HESITANT ARTIST

A good question. My answer is always "Art isn't for everyone." And to force it on clients is unproductive. People of another generation—of the depression era or of the war years—rarely had time for leisure pastimes of this sort and they often see it as merely "kindergarten stuff." It is a difficult viewpoint to reverse. When I know I will have a new client in my group, I plan ahead to ensure a highly successful, perhaps diversional activity. I want to make the client feel like an artist, *feel* that they can be successful before I ask them to take risks. I also do not saturate my group members, instead I try to alternate between heavy-duty emotional or high-risk groups and lighthearted, more relaxing get-to-know-you kind of groups. Also, making sure the process and materials are age appropriate is important. I avoid using crayons, preferring to use the more "artsy" Craypas. When confronted with the "this is kids' stuff" comment, I generally reply with a chuckle and the comment that they should take a look at the local art museum, and say, "We could make a fortune with this!" After that levity, we can discuss the true worth of art . . . Did they enjoy themselves? Did they learn anything?

I have a client with memory loss and confusion related to alcohol abuse. She has been a member of my group for many years and used to tell my interns, "I don't like coming here, but I enjoy it and keep coming back!" She says that she tries to keep herself busy all day so that she does not think about things and then, into my group she comes and is faced with the issues she avoids! The difference is that she can sort through her emotions and issues with friends and peers that understand and support her. She is the biggest advocate for art therapy I know!

WHAT TO DO WITH THE LOWER-LEVEL CLIENTS

First of all, this classification (lower-level) is not meant to demean or label anyone, but is only used in reference to clients with moderate confusion and/or significant physical challenges. There are many treatment plans in this book directed toward that population, and many of the other processes can be adapted to be used on all capability levels. For these groups, personal introspection is less of a focus. Instead, I focus on group dynamics, task completion, color and shape identification, sensory stimulation, and reminiscence. Hand-over-hand task completion is often necessary, as well as much more preparation time; however, the satisfaction on the clients' faces when they see something they created and contributed to being displayed and appreciated by others is always gratifying. If they are significantly confused and do not appear to get much from their involvement in the group, the clients' *families* appreciate their involvement in the creation of art and thier inevitable pride when they take the artwork home to cherish.

WHAT ABOUT LOW-VISION CLIENTS?

It takes a little imagination to do some simple artwork with clients who have limited vision abilities. If they can see colors, blurrily even, perhaps start them out doing loose watercolor paintings of large flower pictures. Relate their work and style to the French impressionists! Limiting the work surface by having them work in a low-rimmed tray works well with both the low-vision client and the confused client because it limits distraction and provides boundaries. Scented markers and paints are a great idea, but are not as rewarding to work with as far as results go and should not be used with confused clients for obvious reasons.

OTHER THINGS TO CONSIDER

Create a reference box that categorizes pictures from magazines into flowers, landscapes, animals, buildings, etc., so that you have immediate resources for studio groups (meaning teaching technique-type groups) and collage works. Also, for any work that is displayed (with permission of course) try to matte the artwork so that it has a more professional presentation. It is great to matte a "beginner's" artwork. It gives it that extra touch and helps beginners feel that the work they do is adult and important. The corporation I work for has a national contest for artistic endeavors. You may decide to have a judged show of your clients' works; however, I feel that in the long run, competition among artists in this setting is not always productive and can lead to resentment among group members. Remember, art for its own sake is its own reward.

The ideas presented in this book have been met with interest and enjoyment by the clients with whom I have worked. I hope that they assist you in opening the windows of imagination and the doors to self-exploration for your clients and yourself.

Chapter 2

Fabric Techniques

A WORD ABOUT WORKING WITH FABRICS

The following processes use a variety of fabric techniques, including collage of various textures and types of fabrics, as well as unique dying techniques such as tie dyes and ink staining. The best thing about using fabric in art therapy is that most of the time it requires you to purchase very few supplies, as fabrics are a common donation item or can be requested as a donation from upholstery shops or fabric stores by asking for end-of-bolt remnants and out-of-production fabrics. Also check with interior design companies for their obsolete sample books!

I like using fabric for some projects not only because of its potential use for "flat" artwork, but also for its ability to be stretched over a frame, or even quilted, depending upon the process and the need for adaptability.

The use of "Tie-Dye Cords" (a product that gives you the dye on a string) and inks give the same effect on fabric as watercolor paints have on paper. They often create beautiful washes and flowing colors spontaneously.

The usefulness of fabric processes with lower-level or sensory stimulation groups is self-evident. It is a trigger of reminiscence for many and provides the opportunity for many visually impaired clients to "see" by feeling.

Fabrics have numerous uses; don't worry if you can't sew a hem . . . Do you own a hot-glue gun?

FABRICS AND PAINTS

A Day in the Life: Medium- to High-Level Cognitive Functioning

This therapy group addresses people's personal philosophies and allows for exploration of shared experiences when dealing with long-term hospitalization or a significant change in lifestyle. The use of "Luma" inks here offers a vibrant interpretation of feelings.

Materials needed: old cotton sheeting (white), cut into 24″ × 36″ squares; "Luma" concentrated watercolor inks (with eye dropper dispensers); table covers; "Slickers" fabric paints in squeeze bottles; newspaper; spray bottles of water; and wood dowels (optional)

1. Cover tables and lay out, over folded newspaper, one piece of material per person. Dispense inks within easy reach of all clients.
2. Begin discussion by talking about the meaning of personal philosophies. Give examples if necessary, e.g., "Treat others as you would have them treat you." Discuss how personal philosophies help us get through hard times and remind us of what is important.
3. Ask each participant to think of a philosophy they have adopted or developed to help them deal with everyday life.
4. With this in mind, ask them to choose colors and to create an abstract image of that philosophy; in other words, use color and shape to imply the meaning and importance of their philosophy.
5. Dampen material with spray bottles of water and instruct clients on the usage of eyedropper inks. "Luma" inks are concentrated color, so once applied a little bit goes a long way when sprayed with water.
6. After backgrounds are established, allow pieces to dry somewhat. Remove saturated newspaper from underneath material and wipe up any excess water.

7. While pieces are drying, begin to discuss philosophies. Ask each individual what philosophy they were thinking of as they created the background, and write this across the material with "Slickers" paint. Ask the clients to express the significance of this philosophy to them. Ask if any of the other group participants believe in the philosophy as well.

When each person has discussed their personal philosophy, allow each piece to dry. Finish off by either sewing pieces together for a philosophy mural, or create personal banners for the participants by hemming each piece and adding a dowel to the top hem (see Photo 2.1 and Photo 2.2).

Facing Challenges: High- to Medium-Level Cognitive Functioning

This process was originally implemented as part of a Thanksgiving workshop that focused on the hardships faced by the Pilgrims and the challenges we all face everyday. The focus of this group was to acknowledge the fact that each challenge we face makes us stronger individuals.

Materials needed: cotton sheeting cut into squares approximately 24″ × 36″; "Luma" inks; "Tie-Dye Cords"; various other fabric paints; spray bottles filled with water; newspaper plastic gloves; table; and clothes coverings

1. Prepare tables with covers and lay each fabric square on top of several sheets of newspaper to help absorb paints and water.
2. Lay out fabric paints, inks, and cords all within easy reach.
3. Ask the clients to think about the journey they have made through life. Have them reflect upon the challenges they have faced and the discoveries they have made about themselves.
4. Using the fabric paints provided, ask the participants to express the idea of their challenges through line and color.

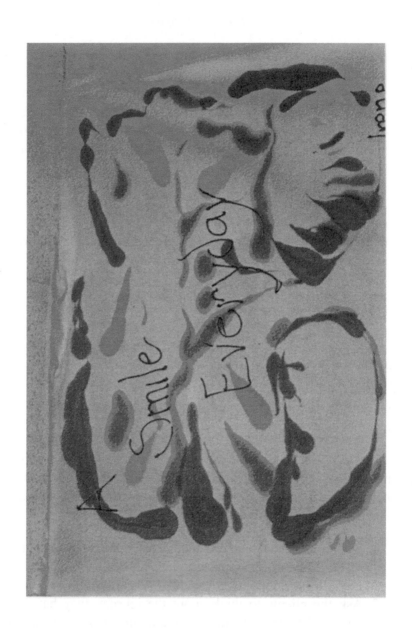

8

PHOTO 2.1 and 2.2. "Day in the Life" Banners

If they are slow to begin, discuss how line and color can reflect emotions and feelings (e.g., red may indicate anger, smooth lines may represent calm).

5. Spray fabric lightly with water to release color in the "Tie-Dye Cords" and to soften and spread the other inks and paints.

6. As individuals are finishing their pieces, encourage them to share their stories with the group, giving enough time and attention to all members. When everyone is finished painting, remove the newspaper and allow the fabric to dry somewhat.

7. Next, ask participants to think about what they have learned about themselves or how they have grown by facing these challenges.

8. Ask them to think of a word that would express that wisdom. Using the "Slickers" paint, have them write that word across their panel. Again, ask them to share their insights with the group.

The finished panels can then be sewn together to form a large wall hanging, or hemmed separately to create personal flags or banners. Displaying their pieces solidifies the experience and serves as a reminder of their personal worth.

Special thanks to Kimberley Galbraith, Recreation Therapist, for her contribution to this process.

Touch Mural: High- to Medium-Level Cognitive Functioning; Low with Adaptations

Human contact—touch—is an important part of our lives. Being touched by others can be affirming, comforting, or therapeutic. Many times, residents in long-term care (LTC) settings do not receive this kind of touch enough. They are touched for repositioning, toileting, and other medical/physical needs, but often miss the benefits of the "caring touch." With this in mind, I developed an art therapy treatment plan to address this issue with both clients and staff.

Materials needed: "Color Switch" fabric paints (these are paints that are heat sensitive); cotton sheeting; 3-D paints ("Slickers"); paintbrushes; and table covers

1. Line tables with covering to prevent paint leakage onto working surface.
2. Lay cotton sheeting on table. Cut fabric to accommodate the number of clients in the group.
3. Set out the "Color Switch" fabric paints and have each client choose a color. Begin the group by discussing the value of touch. Explore the feelings involved with receiving an appropriate human touch. Clients may comment on how it makes them feel cared for and supported.
4. Ask the participants to lay their hands on the fabric. Ask them to help each other trace their hands, with their chosen color, onto the fabric in several places.
5. Using the paintbrushes, the participants fill in each hand-print with that individual's color. As they do this, discuss with them the following questions: Can you ask someone for a caring touch? What would you say? How does an appropriate touch make you feel?
6. The director writes their comments around their handprints on the fabric with the 3-D paint.

When the piece is dry, the clients can then place their hands over another participant's handprint on the mural. As they do this, the colors will change (green turns to yellow, blue to purple, etc.)! Much like the handprints on the cloth, a "warm" touch can bring about unexpected and wonderful changes.

The completed project was hung in a location in my facility where family, staff, and clients pass frequently. I posted an explanation and an invitation to all to place their hand over another's and see what a difference a touch can make.

Adaptations

For lower-cognitive/physical functioning-level clients, use the hand-over-hand method. Assist with tracing and filling in hand-prints. Center focus of group to sensory stimulation, color identification, and one-step directive task following.

"Tie-Dye Cords": Medium- to High-Level Cognitive Functioning; Low with Adaptations

This is a great success-oriented group for those clients who are just beginning to experience art.

Materials needed: "Tie-Dye Cords"; cotton fabric cut into workable squares; water-filled spray bottles set on mist; paper toweling; plastic gloves (optional); scissors; and table and clothes coverings

1. Cover tables and ask participants to cover their clothing. The cords are real fabric dyes, therefore they will permanently stain clothing.
2. Give each participant a square of fabric. Ask them to choose two to three colors of "Tie-Dye Cords." (Assist with identifying the colors, as it can be difficult.)
3. Instruct clients to lay the cords onto the dry fabric in any way they wish.
4. Roll the fabric into a tube with the cords inside.
5. Lay the tube onto paper toweling and saturate both sides with water using the spray bottles. Press the roll down as you spray to encourage color release.
6. Unroll the tube and carefully remove cords. You should have a beautiful repeated design! (See Photo 2.3.)

Once dried, these patterns can be stretched and displayed, or hemmed and used as you would use any colored fabric (pillowcases, scarves, etc.).

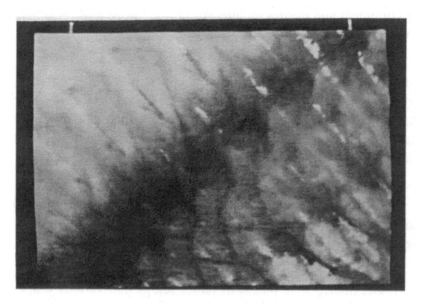

Photo 2.3. "Tie-Dye Cord"

Adaptations

Use the cords on wet watercolor paper to create beautiful watercolor washes and interesting designs. For lower-functioning-level clients, concentrate on choice-making and fine/gross motor skills. Use coffee stirring sticks to drag the cords around paper.

FABRIC/COLLAGE

Sensory Portraits: Medium- to Low-Level Cognitive Functioning; High with Adaptations

The following is an art/tactile stimulation treatment plan that challenges residents, both physically and cognitively, in a group environment and creates an interesting one-to-one tool for others to use.

Materials needed: various colored and textured fabrics (silk, nylon, lace, burlap, leather, tweeds, and artificial fur scraps, etc.); hot-glue gun; one sheet (36″ × 22″) of muslin or other sturdy fabric folded in half, to act as a "base"; stuffing material; and newspapers

Many of the materials needed for this process can be obtained as donations from upholstery shops, interior design studios, or textile merchants.

1. Cut manageable pieces of fabric scraps into various shapes (hand size or slightly larger).
2. Fold "base" material in half and place newspaper between layers to prevent gluing fabric together.
3. Seat clients around a table with fabric within reach.
4. Open the activity with a discussion about what different texture materials are available (e.g., scratchy, silky). Discuss different uses of the various types of fabrics (e.g., flannel is soft, therefore good for pajamas).
5. Pass around the various samples to each member; ask them to identify the kind of material they have and what it would be used for.
6. Next, ask them to pick their favorite fabrics and ask if they, like the fabric, can be soft, scratchy, rough, etc.
7. Ask them to choose a texture and shape they can relate to. (Surprisingly, even our lower-level clients are able to do this!)
8. Then, one by one, instruct them to place their material on top of the base material. Hot-glue the material into place. Repeat with each member of the group.

When all participants have placed their pieces on the base fabric, ask each client to feel the entire collage to experience the different textures. Close the activity by relating how even though fabrics and people are different, when put together, they can create something beautiful and exciting.

We completed the project by sewing together the back and front, and then stuffing and quilting certain areas to give the piece a 3-D effect. The piece of artwork can be used as a one-to-one tool or hung in a client area to provide tactile stimulation to "fidgety" or confused individuals.

Adaptations

Allow higher-cognitive/physical functioning-level clients to both choose a material texture they can relate to and to cut out a symbol, word, or shape to represent them. Continue with the process as outlined above.

Fabric Dolls: Medium- to Low-Level Cognitive Functioning

This process was originally done with a sensory stimulation group of geriatric adults who suffered mild levels of confusion and disorientation. The use of a form of a paper doll made this process immediately nonthreatening to them and enabled them to participate to their potential.

Materials needed: fabric of various sizes, colors, and textures (e.g., corduroy, fake fur, burlap, tweeds) precut into "paper dolls"; a large piece of dark-colored poster board; rubber cement; and black sharpie markers

To make fabric dolls, fold fabric lengthwise into four folds (like a fan). Cut a half doll shape from the folded side. When you unfold the fabric you should have the doll shapes. Make dolls of different shapes and sizes. See Illustration 2.1.

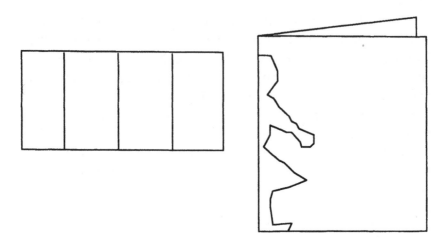

Illustration 2.1. Fabric Dolls

1. Place precut dolls onto table and arrange clients around them.
2. Show the clients the fabric dolls and discuss what they are, and that the forms may represent people.
3. Spend time discussing textures, colors, and the differences between fabrics; e.g., Is this smooth or rough?
4. One by one, ask the clients to pick out their favorite doll and place it anywhere on the poster board.
5. Glue down each doll as it is placed.
6. Show the finished product and explain that they have created not just separate figures, but a *group* of figures.
7. Ask them to tell you things that groups of people do together.
8. Write their answers around the border of the poster board with the marker.

Displaying this piece of artwork is great to remind staff that even the confused and regressed clients still have memories and ideas if given the opportunity and encouragement to respond.

Take My Hand: Medium- to Low-Level Cognitive Functioning

This group activity is designed to combine nonthreatening collage work with discussion for the medium- to low-level LTC clients. It demands hands-on and one-to-one discussion but also offers some group dynamics that are beneficial for any client. Clients are asked to make decisions and to fulfill one-step directives. This process uses fabric scraps from donations made by upholstery stores and interior design companies.

Materials needed: fabric scraps in many solid colors and various textures; black marking pens; scissors; white glue or rubber cement; and heavy poster board or scrap matte board in light colors for background (either one sheet per client or one large sheet for a group project)

1. Cover tables and lay some fabric out within clients' reach.
2. Begin a discussion about hands. Ask the question, "What are some things we use our hands for?" (Picking things up, working, sewing, and touching are good examples.)
3. Ask the clients to reach out and take a piece of fabric. What color is it? What does it feel like? Is it rough or smooth? Pass each client several samples and repeat the questions.
4. Ask them to choose one sample and lay their hand upon it.
5. Trace participants' hands with the marker and cut the shapes out of the fabric.
6. If doing individual projects, ask them to choose a background color and glue the hand onto it. If doing a group project, ask them to take turns gluing their fabric hands onto the community background selected for them.
7. Again, ask "What do we use our hands for?" and write their responses around the fabric hands, adding each contributor's name after his or her quote.

8. Display the finished piece of artwork in the community room or hall.

The Sky's the Limit: Medium- to High-Level Cognitive Functioning

This nontraditional art process involves mostly choice-making by your client(s). The project involves three-dimensional fabric-hanging, so first you must find a way to hang your pieces. Luckily, many facilities have drop ceiling panels, which enable the creative artist to pop the tiles up to tuck fabric underneath. Otherwise, tacking pieces to corner walls will also work to create the 3-D effect desired.

Materials needed: long strips of fabric (twisted, stuffed, tied, or braided, so that the fabric itself is three-dimensional); fabric in 6 foot by 1 foot lengths, if possible (in a variety of colors and textures); step ladder; and tacks

1. Before the group starts, clear space in the room. Directly above that space, mark numbers on the ceiling tiles that are big enough to be seen by the clients. Lay fabric tubes and braids on the floor; circle clients around them.
2. Begin a discussion about the sky. What color is it? Suggest that, as beautiful as the present sky is, wouldn't it be fun to create your own sky?
3. Ask clients to choose a length of fabric that they like, for whatever reason.
4. Ask them to look upward at the ceiling and to choose two numbers.
5. Stretch their fabric from one number to the next, allowing it to hang somewhat off the ceiling.
6. Instruct the next client to choose numbers also; however, his or her fabric must come in contact with the other fabric in

some way. (It could be wrapped around it, crossed over it, etc.)

7. Continue with the entire group. Finish the activity with a community critique of the new sky.

Cloaks: Medium- to High-Level Cognitive Functioning

Cloaks, by definition, are garments made to protect or disguise. They often identify the wearer as a member of a group, such as a warrior or as the member of a royal family.

The following process challenges the artist to create a cloak that defines him or herself in some way. What colors and symbols would the artist use to create a garment of this kind? To complete this group in one session, you will need to spray-paint the cloaks the base color instead of using liquid fabric dyes, or you can predye cloaks in a variety of colors for clients to choose from. By doing this, group time can be used to elaborate on the clients' designs.

Materials needed: old bed sheets (that have been cut into squares, hemmed into a basic "cloak" shape, and gathered at the top with a tie) (one per client); fabric paints; "Tie-Dye Cords" or spray paint (to fill the cloak with a background color); scrap fabric in solid colors of various fabric types; scissors; hot-glue gun; glitter; sequins; and table covers

NOTE: Clients will need plenty of table space to spread their cloaks out while they work!

1. Begin the activity with a discussion of cloaks and their function as described above.
2. Provide cloaks to all participants.
3. Ask the participants to consider what it is that defines them as a person. Invite them to choose a basic color that would reflect something about themselves. They will use this as a

base color. Apply the color using the dye cords (allow a day to dry before moving on) or use spray paint to provide the background color. (You will most likely have to leave the room to perform this task.)

4. While the background color is drying, discuss the possible symbols or shapes that each client would like to use to describe themselves or to indicate what is important to them.
5. Assist with cutting out shapes, if necessary, or include these symbols by drawing them directly on the cloak with fabric paints or markers. Fasten the cut-out shapes with hot glue if necessary.
6. Add sequins or glitter with white glue.
7. When all cloaks are completed and the glue is dried, discuss the markings on each. Ask clients to try them on. Take an instant picture of them if possible.
8. Display the cloaks with an explanation of the process if possible.

"Warm Fuzzy" Group: Medium- to Low-Level Cognitive Functioning; High with Adaptations

The following is a group interaction-based process resulting in two or more wall hangings. This process was originally created with the lower-level client in mind, but could also be used with other populations, with the focus then changing from group interactions and geometric design skills to one-step directive following; color, shape, and texture identifying; and tactile stimulation. Below are directions for both high- and low-level groups. This process uses fake-fur material as a sensory enhancer and dimensional medium.

Materials needed: several large squares of white fake fur (to be used as background pieces) approximately $24'' \times 26''$; several strips of earth-tone colored fur, of various widths that are at least

24″ long; small geometric shapes cut from fur (preferably tan, brown, and black-colored fur of different natural earth-tone); white glue; scissors; and dowels to drape the finished product over (for display)

Use the directions provided here to conduct the activity with a high-level group:

1. Divide group members into smaller subgroups of two to four people. Seat each group around a table upon which lies the 24″ × 26″ background piece of fabric.
2. Discuss the idea of creating a wall hanging together. Explain to participants that together as a group they will create an interesting geometric image. Emphasize that they must decide together how they want the finished product to look, and that they must work together to complete the many physical tasks such as stretching one piece of fabric from one side of the background to the other, as well as placing and gluing fabric shapes.
3. Pass out the supply of fur strips, five to six per group. Ask clients to place and glue the strips to the background. They may use as many or as few as they would like. They may also crisscross pieces if they choose.
4. When done, distribute a variety of geometric pieces to each table (have plenty to pass out). Instruct clients to place and glue these pieces, deciding as a group how and where to place them.
5. Allow 20 minutes for each group to complete its wall hanging.
6. When finished, take time for each group to show off their creation. Discuss how each group came up with a unique image even though they had the same basic materials to use.
7. Ask each group to decide on a name for its work.
8. After all the glue is dried, fold over the top 2″ of the piece and hot-glue a seam to slide the dowel into. Tie a piece of

yarn or string to each end of the dowel and hang the final product.
9. Display the wall hangings with an explanation of each group.

The following directions should be followed to conduct the activity with a low-level group:

1. Using the same materials, distribute strips of fur and assist (hand-over-hand) with placing and gluing the strips in place.
2. After assisting each individual, turn the base piece to help balance the distribution of the materials.
3. Next, provide each member with a geometric shape. One at a time, ask each individual to identify his or her shape. What color is it? Is it soft or rough? Stop frequently to show the other members of the group the progress of the piece.
4. When finished and the glue is dried, ask the clients to run their hands over the entire piece in order to feel the different shapes.

For group levels, this process provides the opportunity to work with a uniquely comforting material. It offers both levels of clients the challenge of working as members of a group while using an often soothing material. The result is not only aesthetically pleasing, but can be used as a sensory stimulation tool in the future. (See Photo 2.4.)

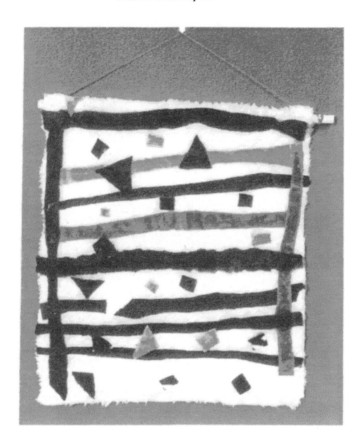

Photo 2.4. "Warm Fuzzy" Wall Hanging

Chapter 3

Paint Techniques

A WORD ABOUT WORKING WITH PAINTS

Painting has many facets that you must consider before you use it with your clients. Can they remember to dip the brush in water, then in paint? Can they identify colors and separate them if they come in a "school pack" palette? Do their hands shake, thereby making the application of paint loose and unrestricted? Is that workable with the process you have chosen to try? Here are some other things to consider:

Watercolors. These tend to bleed and run together unpredictably. Can your client let go of control and adapt to that? If control is an issue with a client or if the client is easily frustrated, you may not want to use watercolors until he or she is comfortable with taking risks.

Acrylics. These have more body and are easily controlled, but application must be precise as they will not blend spontaneously as watercolors will. Acrylics are nice when working with people with visual difficulties, as even the "light" colors are substantial enough to be seen.

Brushes. Stiff brushes should be used when doing detailed work or when using acrylics; fuller brushes can be used for watercolors. Synthetic brushes are good if you don't mind color stains. Personally, I would recommend staying away from camel hair or "cheap" brushes, as many clients find it frustrating and often obsess about loose brush hairs that fall out and end up embedded in their work.

Palettes and water containers. Never use plates or dining cups for paint storage or water storage, as clients will sometimes get confused and drink from them! Instead, use clear plastic containers no higher than five inches tall so that they are able to dip brushes in easily even if they have motor-control problems.

I find it helpful to offer my clients studio group opportunities. This provides them with the opportunity to come into the art room and learn painting techniques and practice with various media so that during their therapeutic group times, they can focus more on feelings and expressions than on the mode of expression. If they are comfortable with the medium, they can come to group with less hesitancy and self-consciousness.

Some of the following processes are geared to the lower-level clients and necessitate more hand-over-hand assistance and direct intervention from the therapist. Sometimes that bothers some professionals; however, I find it acceptable as long as you are assisting clients to fulfill their choices and to enhance their chosen images. In these cases, these are what the goals are: increased self-esteem, decision making, fine and gross motor skills, and reminiscence.

WATERCOLORS

Hidden Images: Low-Level Cognitive Functioning

This process was used with moderately confused clients, with the focus on color selection and challenging abstract thinking. It uses a combination of extra-large, restaurant-size coffee filters and concentrated watercolor inks in eyedropper dispenser bottles to achieve rich colors.

Materials needed: coffee filters (often available in the facility's kitchen); inks in various colors; paper towels; working trays or table covers; spray bottles filled with water; and black permanent markers

1. Distribute filters. Begin a discussion about colors and ask the following questions: What are the colors of the season? What colors are the clients wearing?
2. Assist the clients in folding the filters into fan shapes.
3. Spray each fan with water until well saturated.
4. Ask each client to choose a color. If the clients have difficulty choosing independently, give them a choice between two colors.
5. Hand-over-hand, assist each client with dropping the ink from the eyedropper onto the filter. Ask the clients to choose up to two more colors each. Repeat the hand-over-hand assistance.
6. When all of the clients have applied color to the filters, open the fans to view the color displays.
7. Ask the clients if the colors remind them of anything. Do the forms? Sometimes the vibrant colors are easily recognizable as flower shapes. With encouragement, clients may be able to name flowers of the season. Yellows often are recognizable as sunrises or sunbursts.
8. When the filters are dry, bring them back to the group members and assist them in identifying shapes, such as flowers or butterflies.
9. Outline shapes with the black marker. Use the whole round of the filter or cut the filters in half to limit the focus area.
10. Mount the finished projects on colored poster board or matte board. (See Photo 3.1.)
11. Display each project with the client's name and the title of the work.

The clients not only enjoy working with the vibrant colors, but they continue to gain stimulation from the work when it is displayed in a resident area. By adding the artist's name with the display, other staff are able to give that client positive feedback.

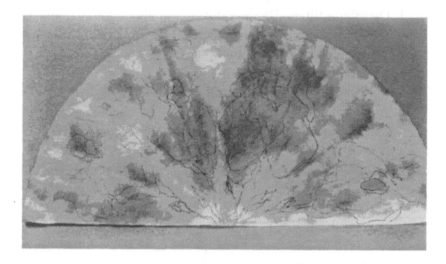

Photo 3.1. Detail from Hidden Images

This process can be done frequently throughout the year, highlighting significant colors of the season.

Resisting Colors: Low-Level Cognitive and Physical Functioning

This process is designed to be used with lower-level clients to provide the opportunity to make decisions and to challenge their ability to think abstractly. The use of concentrated watercolor paints infused on paper is important to the ease of use for these clients. The "Peerless" paint and the appropriate paper are available through most art supply companies and are used primarily for painting on photographs.

Materials needed: watercolor paper cut in small sheets approximately 5″ × 8″ or 4″ × 6″; rubber cement; watercolor paints (such as "Peerless concentrated watercolor paints") and paper torn in pieces; brushes; spray bottles filled with water; working trays; and paper towels

1. Before the group convenes, trickle and flick rubber cement onto the torn pieces of paper to create streaks and dots. Let dry without wiping and make sure the rubber cement is applied generously to create the masking effect you're looking for.
2. Put a tray with prepared paper at each client space.
3. To begin the activity, discuss colors. What are the clients' favorite colors? What colors are they wearing?
4. Spray each client's paper with water. Taking turns, ask each to choose a color. Select that color and apply it to a piece of "Peerless" paper. Assist with placing pieces of shredded paper onto the watercolor paper and distributing the watercolor with the brushes. The paint will resist the areas that the rubber cement has been applied to.
5. Ask the clients to choose another color and apply as before.
6. Allow the paper to dry completely.
7. Rub any residual rubber cement off with your finger tip or an eraser.
8. Looking at the colors and designs, ask the clients if the colors remind them of anything: flowers, sunshine, or anything else? Can they identify the colors on the paper? Can they think of anything else that is the same color?

Matte and display the artwork along with the titles. (See Photos 3.2 and 3.3.) You will find that the colors stay vibrant and provide high contrast to the white of the paper. I like to have mattes prepared before the group so that I can show the clients their work framed and provide them with immediate gratification.

The Passage of Time: Medium- to High-Level Cognitive Functioning

How do we relate to the passage of time? How do we know time moves? We are faced with time every day in many ways: through our clocks and watches (our timekeepers), through the change of seasons and the phases of the moon, the change of the

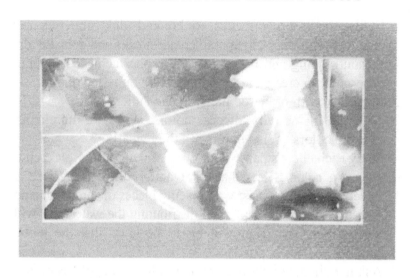

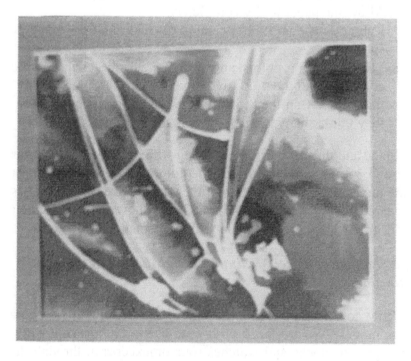

Photos 3.2 and 3.3. Resisting-Color Display

color of our hair, the additional wrinkles to our faces, as well as the additional marks on the wall as our children grow tall. People experience and *feel* time in different ways.

This is a process I did during the change of seasons from summer to fall. The days grow shorter and suddenly we've realized that time has passed. Where did the summer go? It's time now to look at time.

Materials needed: watercolor paper–any size your clients feel comfortable using (11″ × 14″ or so); watercolors (full palette); brushes; water containers; table covers; and quiet music played in background

1. Begin group with a discussion of time (as begun above).
2. Ask clients to paint their vision of the passage of time. It could be abstract or reality-based.
3. Allow 20 to 25 minutes to work quietly.
4. When all clients are done, ask them to share their feelings about time passing.
5. Next ask, "Would you like to stop time? Turn it back? Speed it up?"

The result of this group is generally a serious discussion of mortality and the circle of life we see in nature and in our own lives. Discuss the meaning and usefulness of time lines and the wisdom we have gained as we look back at how we have "spent" our time.

Let It Rain: Medium- to High-Level Cognitive Functioning

This is a quick process that generally generates pleasant rewards due to its "care-less" approach. The process uses the traditional wet-on-wet technique of watercolor painting, paired with a discussion of our feelings about the rain. Use the biggest paper appropriate for the range of motion possible for your clients–smaller sheets of paper for a lesser degree of mobility, larger sheets (18″ × 24″) for greater mobility clients.

Materials needed: watercolor paper; watercolor paints (full palette for each client); concentrated water-soluble inks with eyedropper applicators; metallic paints (if possible); brushes; spray bottles filled with water; paper towels; water containers for each client; and an audiotape of rainstorms (optional but nice)

1. Have all materials laid out on covered tables.
2. Discuss "rain." How do we feel when it rains, physically and mentally? Do we like rainy days? What are the positive aspects of the rain? How does it feel to be caught in the rain? How does it feel to stand in the rain voluntarily? Do we feel drenched or cleansed?
3. Ask each client to create their impression of rain using the materials provided. Demonstrate the wet-on-wet technique. Spray paper, and apply colors loosely, allowing and encouraging them to run together freely without a lot of forethought or predetermination.
4. Ask clients to choose colors that reflect their personal thoughts of rain or rainy days. Spray paper with water.
5. Allow them to work quietly with rain music playing in the background (if provided).
6. When all are done, ask the group if they can guess each artist's feeling about rain from his or her image. Did he or she use traditional "rain" colors (like grays) or bright colors? How does that affect our feelings about rain?
7. Allow the paper to dry flat. Matte and display each artist's "rainstorm."

Color Portraits: High-Level Cognitive Functioning

This is a good introduction to the relationship between color and person. The process follows a discussion of color associations and what our individual color associations are. Discuss colors of passion, anger, happiness, sadness, etc. How do we see these color associations every day (e.g., in advertising, in the clothes we wear, in the colors we choose when we create)?

Materials needed: watercolor paper 8″ × 10″; watercolor paints (full palette); brushes; water containers; and table covers

1. Begin the discussion as mentioned above.
2. Ask clients to create a portrait of themselves using no form, only color. Ask them to choose colors that represent their personalities (how they feel or see themselves). Ask them to use the movement of the color to also indicate something about themselves (e.g., if they are excitable, they may use erratic lines and confetti).
3. Allow 20 minutes to work.
4. When all are finished, ask each artist to share his or her portrait with the group. How would the others describe the artist, based on that person's image? Is this what the artist intended? Could they identify the artist if they hadn't known whose painting was whose?
5. Take turns looking at each individual's work. Do personal color associations come into play here?
6. Display each piece of artwork with a description of the portrait's meaning if permitted by the artist.

Echoes: Medium- to High-Level Cognitive Functioning

This process is based on the "ripple effect." I begin this group with a discussion of how, like a pebble thrown into water, everything we do leaves an effect upon others; things we say "echo," that is, actions ring out from the center of us.

Materials needed: watercolor paper; watercolor paints; brushes; water containers; and black waterproof markers

1. Begin a discussion as indicated above. Ask clients to describe what water looks like after you throw a pebble into it.
2. Ask them to think of something of significance to them and to think of a way to symbolize that. For example, if their freedom is of the most significance, the person may use a bird for a symbol.
3. Instruct them to create their symbol somewhere in the center of their paper with the black marker.
4. Instruct them to create a ripple around it, over and over again until it fills the page.
5. Next, ask them to apply color to the entire page in whatever manner they choose. (They can do a wash over the entire page or separate the ripples by color.)
6. When everyone is finished, ask the group what effect the echo of the image has upon the viewer. Does it make the image stronger? Does it create an idea of the eternity of movements or actions?
7. Display the artwork with an explanation of the process and theory. (See Photo 3.4.)

Master of Art: High-Level Cognitive Functioning

Some cultures believe that to capture an image is to gain control over it. Cavemen, it is theorized, portrayed through cave art the beasts they feared in an attempt to have mastery over them. Other cultures believe to capture a person's image on film is to gain control of their soul. With this in mind, I began this group with a discussion of the artist as master of what they create. Is there a person, situation, feeling, or event we wish we had greater control over?

Materials needed: watercolor paper and paints (full palette); brushes; water containers; and markers

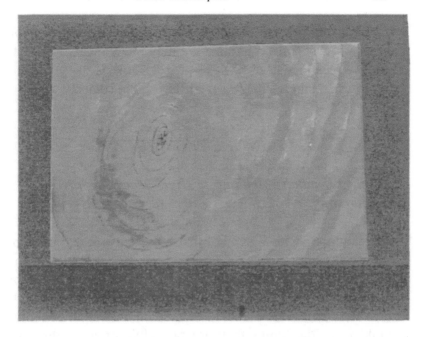

Photo 3.4. Flower Echo: Artist Used a Flower as Her Symbol for Inner Peace and Quietness

1. Open the group with the discussion described above.
2. Ask clients to think of something they wish they had more control over personally or for the good of everyone.
3. Ask them to create an image of that thought. They can represent their idea symbolically or representationally.
4. Allow 20 minutes to complete.
5. Discuss images. Are the ideas they depicted completely out of their control? How can they gain some control over that situation? For example, a client identified the world as a whole as something they wanted control over, specifically to end hunger and violence. How could she make a difference and gain some "control" in the real world? Volunteering was discussed, as well as writing poems or stories that might encourage others to help.

This group has the potential to touch some deeply personal and perhaps volatile emotions. We may never be able to control what we seek to master; however, we can always strive to control ourselves and thereby make the difference to someone else.

PAINTING TECHNIQUES

Repeated Symbols: Medium- to High-Level Cognitive Functioning

Creating a personal symbol that represents something important about us or to us is a powerful thing. Repeating that symbol or incorporating it into a piece of artwork allows us to display ourselves for all to see in a safe, almost anonymous way. In this process, clients are asked to reflect on their individuality–to think of all the things they are–peaceful, strong, wild, afraid, daring, loud (whatever they are is all right)–and then to take that step from internal expression to external realization.

Materials needed: large sheets (22″ × 24″) of watercolor paper (or smaller sheets, depending on the range of motion abilities of your clients); small pieces of poster board (8″ × 11″) to cut a stencil out of; black permanent markers; watercolor paints; brushes; a water container; and scissors

1. Ask your clients to reflect on their personalities as described above. Ask them to embody those traits, or just one of them, into a symbol. For example, if I feel I am a free spirit, I may choose a bird as my symbol.
2. Pass out sheets of poster board and markers. Ask clients to create a *solid* form of their symbol. For example, if a client chooses a symbol with internal markings, such as a happy face, have them just create the outside silhouette of that

symbol on the poster board. They can elaborate on the internal markings later.

3. Cut the symbol out of the poster board to create a stencil or template.

4. Distribute large sheets of watercolor paper. Ask clients to use their template to trace their symbol over and over, starting from the center of the page, until the paper is covered with very little space in between symbols. They can trace in pencil if their hands are shaky, and you can retrace in marker when they are finished. If they have trouble with the tracing, assist with tracing, letting them reposition the template.

5. Once the paper is filled to their satisfaction, ask them to paint the background (the space in between the symbols) with a dark color.

6. When dried, they will elaborate on their symbols with the paints. Ask them to decide if they want each symbol painted identically or differently.

7. When done, ask the clients to share their finished projects with others in the group. What does the symbol stand for? Was it hard to create a symbol to describe you? Was it hard to limit yourself to just one symbol?

8. Title pieces if desired, and display with a note describing the creative process. (See Photo 3.5.)

Distortion for Fun: High-Level Cognitive Functioning

Does the grass have to be green? Does the sky have to be blue? Not in the world of art they don't. Artistic license means control over these things–the sky can be orange, the ocean yellow. In the world of art, we can create anything the way we want it to be.

This process is inspired by an Andy Warhol technique that in a nutshell, repeats a portrait in a series, but manipulates the coloring of each portrait. For this particular group, I surveyed the clients ahead of time and asked them to tell me about a famous

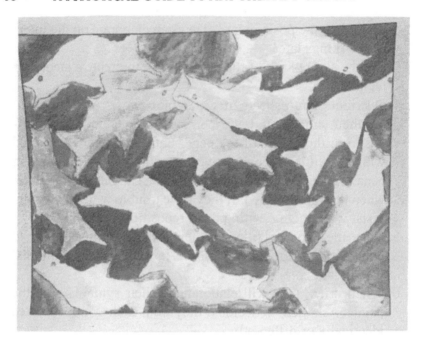

Photo 3.5. Repeated Symbol: "Feeding Frenzy"

person whom they admired. I then found pictures of these people and reproduced them onto 18″ × 24″ sheets of watercolor paper, creating three identical portraits with a black waterproof marker. Then the fun began.

Materials needed: 18″ × 24″ watercolor paper; predrawn portraits (three per client); watercolor paints; brushes; and water

1. Survey clients before the activity, and prepare the series as discussed above.
2. Next, show samples of Andy Warhol's paintings, such as the famous Marilyn Monroe series (easily found at your library).
3. Begin a discussion about freedom in art. Liken the clients to Andy Warhol, and suggest that like him, they can create a whole new look for their admired people.

4. Inform them that the only rule is are that they cannot paint features in realistic colors–faces cannot be black, white, or brown, hair cannot be any of the normal hair colors, etc.
5. Allow enough time for clients to finish all three pictures.
6. When all are finished, ask if the clients found it difficult to break away from realistic coloring in their portrait making. Was it fun or frightening? Most would say it was fun; there always seems to be a lot of laughter with this process.
7. Mount the finished pieces on black poster board and display them as a series. (See Photo 3.6.)

If you have trouble reproducing portraits for this process, feel free to change the focus of the group to something a little less complicated but equally challenging, such as landscapes or animals.

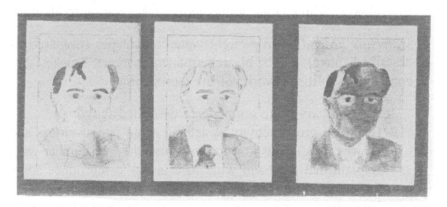

Photo 3.6. Distortion for Fun Shows an Andy Warhol Influence

Old Masters: Medium- to High-Level Cognitive Functioning

Being exposed to famous artists' styles and techniques can be educational and inspiring to artists of many levels. This process combines some art history with the freedom of recreation and group participation. In this group, we enlarge a famous work of art (such as *American Gothic* or *Whistler's Mother)* onto watercolor paper, and separate it according to its content (e.g., man, woman, background elements), and the clients are encouraged to apply color or design as they choose. The clients should not be shown the original artwork ahead of time because it might influence their interpretation of the scene, but they can be given a brief history of the artist or artwork. There are some popular artwork coloring books on the market for kids, which give a brief note on the artwork and the artist, and have very nice black and white linear drawings of paintings. Simply enlarge and reproduce a particular drawing onto watercolor paper to begin this process. Then, cut the painting into sections, keeping in mind the number and ability level of clients you will be working with. For example, a scene may be divided into separate persons, landscape elements, etc., so that you have at least as many pieces as you have clients. With a larger group, work on several reproductions.

Materials needed: heavyweight watercolor paper (prepared as described above); paints; black permanent markers; brushes; and color copies of the artwork you are reproducing

1. Precut artwork into segments as described above.
2. Begin the group activity by talking about famous artists and artwork. Ask clients to name any artists they are familiar with.
3. Explain that they will work as a group to reproduce some famous paintings, only they will add their own touches!
4. Describe the artists that you are reproducing and distribute the pieces based on the ability levels of your clients. For example, you might consider giving a landscape element to a visually impaired client so that he or she won't be frustrated with detailed work.
5. Allow time for all members to complete their contributions.
6. When all are done, assemble the pieces and compare the full picture to the original. (See Photo 3.7.)
7. Give out any more information you have found on the painting's inspiration.

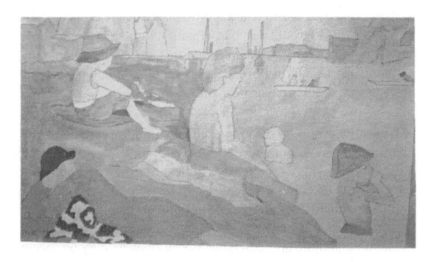

Photo 3.7. Old Masters Collage

I found that although the artists were merely reproducing art-work, they still found personal satisfaction from the group and looked forward to seeing how their creation compared to the original. The final painting was mounted on poster board and displayed along with an explanation of the process.

ACRYLICS

Abstract Art and Randomness: Medium- to High-Level Cognitive Functioning

The purpose of this group is to explore the issues of loss of control that many geriatric individuals, stroke victims, and others feel when hospitalized or admitted into long- or short-term care. The use of abstract-art techniques can demonstrate our ability to face unpredictable situations and to deal with loss of control in a nonthreatening and supportive environment.

Materials needed: prestretched acrylic-primed canvas ($11'' \times 14''$ to $18'' \times 24''$), one per participant; slightly watered down acrylic paints in large containers and in a variety of colors; large paintbrushes ($2''$ utility size); large spoons; small paper cups; newspapers; clothes coverings; and water buckets

Begin the group by discussing the meaning of "random"; i.e., haphazard chance, without definite aim, purposeless, unpredictable, aimless, without thought. Ask them to explore what random things affect us (such as weather conditions). Discuss how random and unpredictable relate. What unpredictable things affect us (such as health matters)? Then talk about how we deal with the random and the unpredictable. Some answers may be "acceptance" or "try to adapt." Finally, explain how, with paints, colors, and random distribution of lines, the concept of randomness can be expressed on canvas.

1. Cover the floor with newspapers.
2. Lay canvases on the floor, leaving enough space between materials for splash during paint application.
3. Have a variety of colored acrylic paints in large containers within reach, along with brushes, spoons, and cups.
4. Lead participants through instruction or a demonstration of how to apply paint to the canvas by throwing, splashing, and pouring the paint. Ask them to try *not* to purposefully create an image, but just to allow the unpredictable to occur.
5. Ask clients to finish their pieces; allow them to watch others until all clients are finished.
6. Afterwards, ask what things were going through their minds as they worked. Were they satisfied with the results of their works? Did they try to create something recognizable to others? Were they able to just let go of their thoughts and just take pleasure in the freedom the process implied? At this time, issues of control may arise from the participants

and a discussion on how, when approached in the right way, the unpredictable can be dealt with in a positive manner.

7. Display the projects together as a mural or individually, with titles designated by the artists.

Music can really be a factor in how the pieces are created; for example, slow, quiet music played during this experience may cause more somber effects than more cheerful, upbeat music.

Repeat Yourself: Medium- to High-Level Cognitive Functioning

What happens when you repeat yourself? You gain people's attention, you give that comment or word additional strength, you mark it as something extra important. That is the basis for this process, which asks participants to choose a word that is especially important for them and to repeat it in many different forms in a word and color collage. This is a good activity to use as an introduction to art therapy because it requires no "classic" art skills, yet introduces them to art media and the group process, as well as helps the group members get to know each other by learning what is *really* important to each. Our society needs rules to feel safe. At least there are no rules in art.

Materials needed: watercolor paper (12" × 15" or bigger, depending on the gross motor skill level of your group); acrylic paints (full palette); table covering; water containers; and brushes

1. Discuss the purpose of "repeating yourself" (as explained above).
2. Ask each person to think of one particular word that holds significance to him or her. (You might ask the group a question such as, "What's important in your life?")
3. Encourage clients to think of a color that they feel would be appropriate to their particular word and instruct them to use

it as their background color. (This could be done in watercolor also.)

4. Next, ask them to express their word over and over again, in
   lettering of different sizes, forms, directions, acrylic-paint
   colors, etc. on the paper.
5. Allow 20 to 30 minutes to work and ask members to share
   their work with each other. Ask why each client's word is
   important to him or her? Does seeing it repeated over and
   over give it more power, or does it weaken it? Display the
   finished products if the group allows. A wall of important
   words, repeated, is reason to pause and consider the people
   behind those words.

Rules: High-Level Cognitive Functioning

This is an interesting process involving the participants in an
active discussion and clarification of their feelings regarding
rules. If your clients are in some kind of institution (day treatment centers, hospitals, or health or rehabilitation centers), suddenly they are finding their lives governed by rules created by
others–strangers who have no real connection to them. This situation increases the feelings of loss and anger clients in those
circumstances may feel. This group activity provides a chance to
really examine rules, determine what they are and how they
function, and to determine their positive and negative influences
in our lifestyles.

Materials needed: prestretched canvas (primed for acrylic paints
if feasible) or heavyweight watercolor paper; acrylic paints in a
variety of colors; brushes of various sizes; water containers; and
table covers

1. Begin a group discussion of rules. What kind of rules are
   there? There are internal rules ("This is wrong or right
   because I feel it . . .") and external rules ("Stop at the red

light"). How do rules make you feel? (Some will like rules, some won't!) How does breaking the rules feel? Ask each person to define their feelings regarding rules.

2. Using the paints provided, ask clients to choose a color and a pattern to cover their entire sheet of paper. Explain to clients that their choice should reflect their personal feelings about rules. For example, if a client likes rules and rules make him or her feel comfortable, the client may paint a solid, warm color as his or her background. If the client doesn't like rules and feels rules are controlling, he or she might paint a background in black, resembling jail bars.

3. Allow the work to dry for a few minutes and then ask clients to consider life without rules. What would that feel like? How can they portray that using colors and lines?

4. Ask them to create that feeling right over their existing painting, but not to cover it completely. For example, our jailed person may paint dreamy clouds over or between his/her bar cells.

5. When all are through, ask them how they think rules, or the lack thereof, coexist together.

Chapter 4

Clay Techniques

A WORD ABOUT WORKING WITH CLAY

Claywork is difficult and rewarding for many clients because of its tactile and physical nature. The artist definitely needs good hand strength to work with this medium independently; however, most of the time the therapist, if allowed the prep time, can prepare the medium in some ways, such as rolling out slabs ahead of time, thereby allowing the client time to create without the frustration and physical demands.

The following processes were done with regular fire clay (as opposed to no-fire or oven-fire clay). If you don't have a kiln in your facility, many ceramic supply stores rent space in their kilns. Some clays do have toxic ingredients, so make sure you review any safety data sheets that come with your purchase.

Some clients dislike working with clay because of its messy qualities. You can supply them with rubber gloves or just encourage them to believe that to be messy is to be artistic!

CLAY

Masks: Medium- to High-Level Cognitive Functioning

Halloween naturally reminds us of wearing masks and costumes; however, creating masks at any time can express the thoughts, hopes, and fears of the creator. In story and legend, masks were used by individuals either attempting to disguise themselves or taking on the identity or spirit of someone or something else. The following treatment plan places the mask-making process in the historical context of legends and rituals of many cultures. It also gives groups the chance to glimpse the inner spirit of the artist through an interpretation of his or her outer self.

Materials needed: speckled red Indian clay (for kiln) or terra-cotta "Ovencraft II" clay (which can be baked in an oven); one ceramic art mask for each participant (average cost: $7.00) to use as a mold (or paper maché art masks, if cost is inhibitive); a rolling pin; plastic forks; plastic wrap; paper towels; ceramic carving tools; sponges; and water containers

Before the group activity begins, wrap mask forms with plastic wrap. Roll out pieces of clay into slabs about one-quarter inch to one-half inch thick, and drape over mask forms. Mold the mask with your hands so that each participant has a good facial form with which to begin their project.

NOTE: Do this ahead of time to allow the group time to be spent on the actual creative aspects of mask-making rather than on the mechanics of it. If your group time is longer than the 45 to 60 minutes that I had allotted, and/or your clients are more physically able, by all means, include them in the physical techniques of clay work. Lightly spray masks with water and cover in plastic until group time.

1. Pass out clay masks.
2. Introduce the subject of masks. Can they be a disguise? Discuss tribal or native beliefs and customs. Explore the wearing of masks during celebrations or rituals, sometimes done to express "animal spirits," or as a part of telling a

story involving legendary gods or characters. (Do some library research!)

3. Ask each client to consider some aspect of themselves that they feel is important. Ask them to then think of some way to express that aspect in their treatment of the mask in front of them. Ask them to make the mask an *extension* of themselves. It should reveal something about them to the viewer—reflect who they are, how they see themselves, or what is important to them. Here is an example: My client saw herself as being trapped. Her mask turned her into a pilot, with a scarf blowing across her neck. This represented her desire for freedom and control, not necessarily expressing who she was, but what she wanted and what was important to her.

   If clients have a difficult time getting started, ask them individually, "What kind of person are you?" At this phase of the process, each individual or group may use this opportunity in a different way. Go with it; that is, encourage clients that no mask can be wrong, no interpretation of the idea can be wrong. Instinctively, the client will share with the other members of the group what he or she feels is appropriate.

4. Make sure each person has carving tools and extra clay to assist with the creation of the mask.

5. Invite them to consider the area surrounding the face of the mask. Also, the "hair" area can be a great opportunity to be creative!

6. Instruct clients to use water and sponges to give the mask a smooth finish if desired. NOTE: This whole process is done with the clay draped over the mold for stability and form.

7. When clients are finished (give about 20 minutes), ask them to share their thoughts about their creations. What can the other members of the group tell about the artist? Do their

thoughts reflect the artist's concept of his or her own piece? Were there things they tried to convey in the mask that they had difficulty creating in the clay?

8. Instruct clients to make holes at the top of their masks (to later hang with string or rope).
9. Ask the group members if they enjoyed themselves and if they learned anything new about themselves or each other.
10. Allow the masks to dry slowly *on the molds.* Cover loosely with plastic wrap. When they reach a leather-hard state, remove them from the mold. Again, cover loosely and let dry slowly so that they do not crack. Remember, the mold *must* be removed before firing or baking.

Display the masks in their raw terra cotta form, along with a description of the process and some quotes from the members of the group regarding their pieces. The display serves as a reminder that no matter our age or abilities, we all still have hopes and beliefs about ourselves, and we still struggle to look under our masks and see our true inner spirit.

Nuts and Bolts: Medium- to High-Level Cognitive Functioning

This process came about after a discussion about "holding it all together." "Holding it together" is more difficult at some times in our lives than at others; demands are made of us in different degrees and we either feel we can juggle these demands or be pulled apart by them. The group activity pairs clay (a malleable substance) with metal nails, screws, nuts, and bolts, and looks at external ways for us to symbolically hold ourselves secure.

Materials needed: red terra-cotta clay or regular hand-building clay; a kiln for firing; clay tools and texture devices; nuts; bolts; nails; screws; rolling pins; table covers; and water

1. Begin a discussion about the purpose of nuts, bolts, and screws. (For example, they hold things together, make things more secure, make things sturdy, etc.)
2. Give each person a small lump of clay.
3. Ask them to think of something in their lives that could use a little reinforcing and to imagine that something as having a shape. Ask them to create that shape or symbol from the clay. They can make it three-dimensional or roll their clay out into a slab and cut it.
4. Instruct them to use the nails, bolts, etc., to pierce the clay form. The nails can pierce, the nuts and bolts can come together after piercing the form, or they can simply be pushed into the clay.
5. When clients have finished, ask them to describe what their symbols represent. Does the presence of the metal objects seem to make that image stronger? (For example, I had a client who suffered from severe arthritis pain in her hands. She traced her hand into the clay and used the nuts and bolts as joints to replace the suffering natural joints in her hands.)
6. Fire the objects at their normal firing temperature. The metal parts will turn black and provide an interesting color contrast to the red clay. There is no need to glaze the bisqueware.

At the next meeting, return the objects to their creators as a reminder of their personal ability to "hold things together."

Chapter 5

Collage Techniques

A WORD ABOUT WORKING WITH COLLAGE MATERIALS

"Collage" is a French word meaning, among other things, "clean out your supply cabinets." This artform, because it brings together many diverse components, offers a wide variety of inspiration and expression possibilities.

In the following process, you will use organic objects and modern machinery, glitter, feathers, mirrors, doorknobs, jars, and scraps of matte board and poster board. Although collage techniques are mess-intensive—all those supplies!—they provide more opportunities to truly reflect ourselves in our creations. What are the differences between a glitter "person" and a bark "person"? What motivates a client to choose a brick pattern instead of a Band-Aid℠? These are things you will find out when you offer this variety of materials for self-expression.

Many of these techniques mention the use of a hot-glue gun. This is meant to be used by the therapist and never the client. Every person I know who has used a hot-glue gun has inevitably burned themselves to some degree, and most of the client populations you are working with are not familiar enough with the tool to use it safely. You are not impeding their independence by being safety conscious, and hot glue is an immediate fixative used to keep the creative process moving along. Many of the supplies used are scavenged from staff and donations, so always be thinking creatively when offered the unusual.

COLLAGE

Copy Machine Art: Medium- to High-Level Cognitive Functioning

In order to introduce clients to "modern technology," I used the facility copy machine to demonstrate photography techniques. Many items were supplied for clients to choose from in order to create a picture of themselves through collage. Once the actual xeroxing was done, participants colored their creations by hand. The finished product was comparable to hand-painted black-and-white photographic efforts.

Materials needed: a copy machine (preferably a machine on wheels so that you can take it into your group room for this process); a variety of natural and man-made objects (e.g., bark, patterned fabric, books, flowers, feathers, cotton balls); a plain-textured (cotton) white sheet; and colored pencils

1. Orient clients to the copy machine. Describe it as a camera that takes pictures of items placed on the tray.
2. Ask the clients to pick items that might somehow represent themselves or their interests. Explain the process as "creating a collage portrait."
3. Once items are chosen, have the participants lay their objects on the copy machine glass delicately. (Inform clients that the glass surface scratches easily.) NOTE: Remember that items should be placed *face down* as objects are copied from the bottom!
4. Lay the white fabric over the items and press in softly around objects that are three-dimensional. This reduces the shadows around these objects and creates better definition.
5. Have the client push the COPY button. Encourage clients to experiment a bit with the machine. For example, an individual could do three copies of the same setup and easily create a "series."

6. Remove items and continue with each member of the group.
7. Next, ask the creators to choose special areas that they would like to highlight. Demonstrate that light application of colored pencil, even over gray areas, effectively draws attention to details.
8. When the clients are finished, ask members of the group to identify the creator of each collage by the characteristics he or she chose to use in the collage. (See Photo 5.1.)

You can also have the participants include personal objects or photographs in their collage. Many clients include their own hands as an identifying factor in their piece, with outstanding results! You might want to follow the activity with a discussion about how

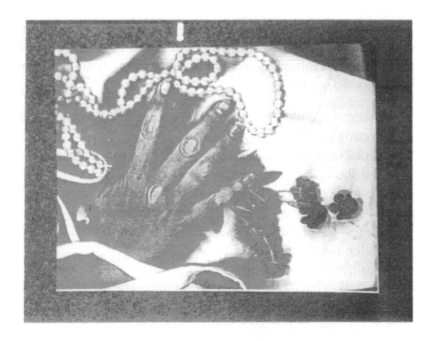

Photo 5.1. Copy Machine Art Collage

individuals may have the same objects in their creation, yet the meanings may be different.

Objects of Art: Medium- to High-Level Cognitive Functioning

This process challenges higher-level-functioning clients to consider abstract symbolic concepts. Each client is given an item that they must interpret and incorporate into a painting. Before the group begins, the leader will bring up the topic of "multisymbolic images"; that is, objects that have abstract or poetic meanings besides their normal definitions. For example, a key is traditionally a piece of metal that fits a lock and is needed to unlock or lock something. Another interpretation of a key could be a magical object that can lock or unlock parts of another person's spirit or memories.

Materials needed: This process requires you to be somewhat of a scavenger, looking for objects in a variety of sizes and possible meanings. The following is a list of suggestions along with possible "poetic" meanings:

- Brick: to build, to create, to provide the foundation, to destroy (e.g., throwing a brick)
- Clock or watch: a timekeeper, shows the passing of time
- Tree branch: family tree, growth
- Driftwood: being carried away, affected by nature
- Eyeglasses: being able to see more clearly
- Shoes: travel, filling someone else's shoes
- Ruler: measuring up
- Feather: freedom, flight
- Adhesive bandage: to cover a wound, to heal and protect
- Eraser: to fix mistakes
- Yo-yo: ups and downs
- Chain links: keeping something secure, bound up
- Compass or map: finding your way, not getting lost

- Doorknob: allowing you to open or close doors
- Flag: loyalty, allegiance
- Hat: prestige, authority, protection from the elements
- Toy spider: something scary, mysterious
- Lightbulb: ideas, creativity, intuition

Other materials needed: 12″ × 15″ poster board; acrylic paints; brushes; water containers; and hot-glue gun

1. Begin the group activity with all items placed on the table within easy reach of the clients.
2. Open a discussion of objects' possible multiple meanings and perhaps discuss how symbolic meanings are often given to common objects or things in poems and songs.
3. Select several objects and see if the clients can assign poetic meaning to these objects.
4. Next, ask each client to choose an object they feel they can relate to. Inform them that they will incorporate that poetic meaning into a painting/collage, using that actual object.
5. Distribute materials.
6. Hot-glue the objects where clients place them on their boards.
7. Allow 20 to 25 minutes for clients to work on their pieces.
8. When everyone is finished, ask them to share their work with the group along with their poetic interpretation of the object.
9. Ask the other members of the group if they have a different interpretation of the objects.

This is a fun and enlightening process for many reasons. The clients will be working with three-dimensional objects of various weights and textures and will probably find it challenging to incorporate the actual object into an otherwise flat painting. The finished products are interesting to view and they open the door for discussions among the clients. One client of mine chose the doorknob because she felt trapped and wanted to have control over her comings and goings. The rest of the group discussed the other meanings of opening doors–to the imagination, to creativity, etc.–and also discussed different kinds of freedoms.

Don't be afraid to introduce your clients to the unconventional. Sometimes they embrace it.

Aliens: Medium- to High-Level Cognitive Functioning

This process challenges clients' creativity and sense of fun by allowing them to create an "alien" using precut shapes of various colors. It involves both motor skills and imagination, and allows for introspection in a nonthreatening context.

Materials needed: matte poster board scraps cut into various geometric and odd shapes in a variety of colors and sizes (keep in mind, you will need shapes for head parts, body parts, legs, arms, and eyes, so provide a wide selection); artificial feathers in bright colors; patterned paper cut into small shapes; glitter; white glue; clear tape; and scissors

1. Distribute poster board materials. Make sure each person has a variety of "body parts" within their reach.
2. Explain to clients that they are about to discover and create a new breed of creature; they may create it in any way they like: scary, friendly, big, little . . . whatever they want. They can use the materials provided to create the body, and they can embellish the alien with the other items when done.
3. Ask them to piece together the body, assisting them to tape the parts together from the back, if necessary.
4. Next, distribute the rest of the supplies. Assist with gluing or taping the additions in place.
5. When clients are finished, ask them to introduce their creations to the group. Ask clients to name their aliens, if possible. Ask each client to tell the group about his or her

alien. Is it happy or fierce? Does it like other people? Is it
strong? What does it do? Is it a leader or a follower?
6. Ask the group to come up with a name for the collection of
   aliens? Where might they have come from? What is their
   history?
7. Invite clients to take their new companions home with them.

This group can be highly successful, providing an aesthetically pleasing image as well as providing an outlet to discuss the
clients' own fantasies or fears in the guise of their new creation.
The use of brightly colored materials helps keep the group light,
fun, and nonthreatening. If your group members can handle more
items, you could also include old jewelry, buttons, and zippers,
all hot-glued into place.

Matte Mosaics: Low-Level Cognitive Functioning

The following treatment plan is ideal for a low-level group, as
it focuses on fine and gross motor skills, decision making, color
and shape identification, and group dynamics.

This process calls for a product called "railroad board," which
is similar to matte board in weight. I recommend this weight
instead of poster board because participants can handle it more
easily; if you have scrap matte board available to you, use it!
Heavier boards allow for the participants to feel as well as see
their creation when through. This technique can also be done
with black poster board and colored construction paper, but you
lose the tactile benefits that handling weightier items bring. The
finished product is aesthetically pleasing and shouldn't result in
the dreaded "that's for little children" comment you may get
from staff and other clients. The displayed product is also useful
to other staff when interacting with those clients by providing
them the opportunity to further reinforce the basic knowledge of
color and shapes at any time.

Materials needed: an 18″ × 24″ sheet of black railroad board; hot-glue gun; and geometric shapes cut from various colors of railroad board or matte board

1. Place the shapes on the table within reach of clients.
2. Spend time reviewing the shapes. Ask each individual to hold the shape. Can they tell you what color it is? Can they think of something else that is that color or shape? (If that client cannot answer, ask for help from the rest of the group.)
3. Place several pieces of different sizes, shapes, and colors directly in front of the clients.
4. Using one-step directives, ask them to pick a shape, identify color and shape, and place it on the black surface.
5. Assist with applying glue, or tack the shape on with the hot-glue gun. (Note: Always keep the hot glue away from participants!)
6. Continue taking turns to place shapes on board until the surface is well covered. (See Photo 5.2.)

Black is best for the background color for the board, as it makes applied shapes and colors easier to see for those whose vision is limited.

The Best of You: High- to Medium-Level Cognitive Functioning; Low with Adaptations

Self-criticism is an easy habit to fall into. It is much easier to look at ourselves and see our faults than it is to see our beauty. We are often embarrassed to self-compliment because we don't wish to be thought of as vain or braggy; however, taking a less critical look at ourselves is an important step in self-acceptance. Self-acceptance is necessary for us to flourish, and highly important to clients in a long-term care or rehabilitation setting where they are challenged constantly and have the opportunity to dwell on

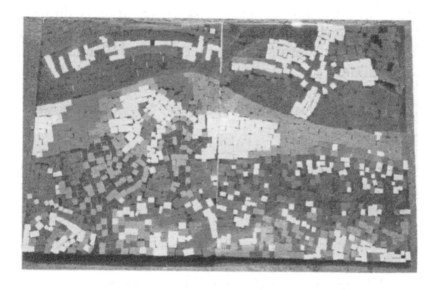

Photo 5.2. Matte Mosaic: Desert Cactus Collage

their "shortcomings." There comes a time when we have to stop worrying about supposed vanity and concentrate on self-love. What follows are two treatment plans based on the same issues, but adapted for different level-functioning clients.

Materials needed for a high-level group: 35mm camera with adjustable focus; black-and-white film; colored pencils; and an available copy machine

Materials needed for a medium- to lower-level group: precut pictures of body parts (e.g., eyes, nose, mouth); glue sticks; and colored construction paper

1. For both groups, begin a discussion of self-criticism. Talk about how we are often too critical of ourselves, often seeing and pointing out our shortcomings and less-than-attrac-

tive features to others. Ask clients if it is difficult to acknowledge the good in themselves without seeming vain?

2. Ask them next to think of themselves less critically and to identify one physical feature of themselves that they think is attractive or that they are pleased with. Be prepared for anything here; I had a client who thought his feet were his most attractive feature!

3. Ask each person to tell the others what personal feature they like best and why. In my experience, the other group members will support the client's choice with compliments and attention.

Continue with the following instructions for a *high-level group:*

4. Using the camera, take a close-up picture of each client's chosen feature. This can be best done with a manual-focus camera, which will allow you to take unconventional shots of the features at close range. (Autofocus cameras won't let you get that close.)

5. End the group and get pictures developed before the next meeting. Enlarge the pictures on the copy machine to approximately 8″ × 10″ if possible, or take them to a professional printing shop and have them run copies for you.

6. At the next meeting, distribute the photocopies and ask participants to highlight their photocopied features with a light application of colored pencil. NOTE: Even coloring over dark gray tones adds interest to a black-and-white copy.

7. Display the pictures.

With the high-functioning group, you could give them several copies of the same picture, and they could imitate an Andy Warhol print technique by using unusual colors on each picture and displaying them as a series!

Use these directions for *low-level groups:*

4. Ask the clients to pick out their selected feature from the collage pictures provided. Instruct them to choose a variety of pictures of the same feature, in a variety of sizes, to fit onto a 5″ × 7″ piece of paper.
5. Using the glue sticks, help them to glue the pictures onto the paper.
6. When clients are finished, ask them to show their work to the rest of the group. Determine if anyone else shares that feature. (For example, ask, "Did anyone choose eyes?" and "How are your eyes different from someone else's?")
7. Display or let clients take the pictures back to their rooms as a reminder of the group's purpose and for stimulation.

All of Me: Medium- to High-Level Cognitive Functioning

This process requires a life-size body silhouette that you will cut into pieces equal to the number of people in your group. You don't want them to guess what the "puzzle" will be until you start putting it together, so cut the pieces into irregular shapes; disguise the more recognizable features by making them less realistic and a little more abstract. Once pieces are cut associate words with those parts and assign the artist the correct associations to work from. For example, give the artist with the head piece a slip of paper that says "thoughts, dreams." Foot people get "stability, movement"; torso people get words like "heart, center"; arms people get "reaching out, providing"; etc.

Materials needed: body silhouette cut from poster board or heavy watercolor paper; slips of paper with word associations; acrylic paints; brushes; markers; crayons; water containers; and masking tape

1. Begin the group activity by telling your clients that they will be creating a puzzle. Have clients choose a puzzle piece.

2. Next, hand each client the slip of paper that relates to the body part he or she has chosen.
3. Instruct the clients to each create an image that somehow reflects the ideas written on their paper. It can be abstract or representational. Allow 20 minutes to work.
4. Beginning with the head piece, ask the artist what word he or she had and to describe how he or she created the image. Tape the head piece to the wall.
5. Continue assembling the puzzle in a logical order (neck, torso, arms, etc.).
6. When complete, look at the final image. What other associations can clients make with the body parts? Do they differ from what you selected for them?
7. Discuss the fragmentation of the body and the reunion of it. Does this relate to the group members? If they could have knowingly chosen a part to create, what would it have been? Does this reflect their perceived role in the group? Their personality?
8. End the activity by having clients name their creations.

Mirror, Mirror: Medium- to High-Level Cognitive Functioning

What is the purpose of a mirror? It reflects our outer selves, what we look like to others. This process matches outside reflections with the opportunity to create a more important reflection of our *inner* selves. The variety of collage materials available to your clients is very important here so that they can more specifically represent what they are truly like on the inside.

Materials: precut matte boards, in a variety of colors, to serve as frames around craft-store mirrors (one per client); collage materials such as feathers, glitter, fabrics, paints, and white or hot glue

I discourage the use of magazine pictures for this activity because the result should be a reflection of the artist, not someone else's perception and images.

1. Lay out all materials on tables.
2. Begin a discussion of mirrors as reflective devices. How do mirrors "judge" us? Do they cast a complete image of who we are?
3. Ask participants to choose a precut frame. Offer several colors to choose from.
4. Ask them to use the collage materials to assemble images of themselves that would best reflect their *inner* selves.
5. Allow approximately 20 minutes to complete.
6. When complete, affix a mirror inside each frame.
7. Ask members to share their reflections with each other. Do they feel, by looking at their mirrors, that they see a more complete image? What can the other group members see about that individual from their frame? Did the artist create an image to portray his or her true self or who he or she wants to be or become? (See Photos 5.3 and 5.4.)

Dream Bottles: High- to Moderate-Level Cognitive Functioning

Having a dream or goal is an abstract activity most of us participate in. We think of it, build the course of our lives around it, strive toward it, and yet it continues to be "out there," an abstract thought without form.

The following process acknowledges our dreams and goals and gives them form. By giving them form, we give them weight and substance and provide ourselves with a concrete focal point to remind us of the beauty of that goal. Goals are important to everyone, especially to people in health care or rehabilitation settings. Be aware that the discussion of dreams and goals could be upsetting to some clients who may feel their goals are out of

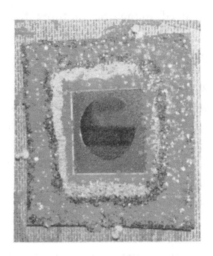

Photo 5.3. Mirror, Mirror Project Where the Artist Reflects His/Her Exuberance Toward Life by Using Glitters

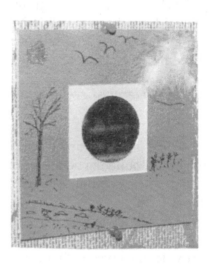

Photo 5.4. Mirror, Mirror Project of a More Quiet and Reserved Individual

reach, and be prepared to offer support and optimism. Our dreams may change throughout our lives. Our expectations change, but the value of dreams stays the same: to give hope and direction.

Materials needed: clean and empty clear glass jars (or plastic, depending on your population) in a variety of sizes from 20 ounces to very small jelly jars (have several available so each client has many choices); "Glitter Strings" (metallic twist ribbons in gold and iridescent colors) untwisted and cut into small pieces; various metallic and pearlized papers (cut or torn into strips); small white strips of paper (one per client) clear tape; and labels for jars (write on each label "dream bottle")

All materials listed will be available through any fine-arts store or craft shop.

1. Discuss dreams, goals, and ambitions as described above. Do we all have a dream?
2. Ask each client to think of a dream or goal that he or she has and write it on a white strip of paper.
3. Instruct each client to choose a jar and to place his or her strip of paper, with the dream written on it, in the jar.
4. Now, ask clients to imagine what giving their dream/goal substance and life would look like.
5. Distribute the rest of the materials.
6. Instruct the clients to use the materials to fill their jars with the "beauty of their dreams."
7. When they are finished, attach the labels to the jars and cover the top with a square of the twist ribbon and a rubber band in the old-fashioned "jelly jar" style.
8. Next, ask clients to share what their dreams are. If they feel comfortable, ask them to pass their jars around to the other group members so everyone can get a closer look.

You will notice that some clients will make certain that the slip of paper that has their dream written on it will be visible, while others will bury their dream beneath the glitter and ribbons. Our dreams are private, sometimes seemingly unachievable, but that never should tarnish the beauty of the dream. These jars are to be a reminder that any dream is beautiful and should never be far from our thoughts.

Spring Collage: Medium- to Low-Level Cognitive Functioning

April is the beginning of spring for those of us around the country who have the privilege of the change of seasons. It is a time that many of us look forward to with much delight and excitement, waiting for the greens and blooms of spring to cheer us. It is also a time that provides a great opportunity to talk color, along with all the things that spring means to both our high-level and low-level clients.

The following process can be used with both levels of clients with adaptations and different levels of complexity. As an introduction to the group, begin talking of spring. With the higher-functioning clients, show pictures of some of the French impressionists' artwork related to flowers, such as Monet artwork. Discuss how Monet shows *areas* of colors rather than each petal and bloom of a spring scene. Take note of the colors used and the way they are applied. The goals here are exploring art history, as well as developing fine motor skills and abstract thinking. For the lower-level group, the goals are more related to reality orientation, fine motor skills, task response, and social interaction. Discuss the colors of spring, the chores they have to complete as part of spring cleaning, and what they remember most about spring.

Materials needed: clear contact paper cut into sheets approximately 8″ × 10″ in size (two per client); colored tissue paper; masking tape; black markers; and working trays (could be the trays their meals come on, or box tops approximately 11″ × 17″ in size with a low lip around the edge)

For lower-level group, pretear tissue ahead of time into irregular pieces at least 1″ × 1″ in size. Before the group begins, take sheets of contact paper and peel away the protective backings. Place one sheet, sticky side up, on each working tray and tape around the borders with masking tape so that the contact paper stays in the trays without lifting up. Set the other unused sheets aside.

1. Begin a discussion as described above. Show reproductions of Claude Monet's paintings to give clients color ideas.
2. Pass out a variety of appropriate spring-colored tissue paper.
3. Ask the artists to choose colors they feel are appropriate. Rip the paper into small pieces for collage technique. (For the lower-level group, use preripped pieces.)
4. Next, pass out the prepared trays to each person.
5. Instruct them to fill the entire sticky area with spring colors by laying pieces randomly over the surface.
6. When the clients have finished, take the other sheets of contact paper, remove backings, and lay them over the tissue collages carefully, pressing to remove bubbles. Remove both sheets from the trays and trim edges.
7. If clients are able, ask them to use the black markers to outline flower designs that they see in their creations.

These may then be hung in a window, as light will shine through the tissue to make a "sun catcher," or they may be matted and displayed. You may even choose to write some of their comments regarding spring directly over the collage. If you choose to display the artwork, add a descriptive note to the display regarding the discussion that occurred during the art making. Maybe you'll inspire more discussion of springtime by others!

Geometric Design: Medium- to Low-Level Cognitive Functioning

Art making is generally considered difficult, if not impossible to do, with clients who struggle with a short attention span, confusion, physical challenges, or dementia. Clients with these problems can gain benefits from the stimulation and positive feedback as long as the process is planned to consider their needs. The results of these sessions can be equally pleasing for client and family with a little extra preparation from you.

The following treatment plan is ideal for this type of group, because it focuses on fine and gross motor skills, decision making, color and shape identification, and group dynamics.

Hot glue, as opposed to white glue, is to be considered here, as hot glue offers you the ability to give immediate feedback to the client by holding up the board as the work progresses. White glue can be messy and must have time to dry before the object can be displayed.

Materials needed: an 18" × 24" sheet of black railroad board; white glue or a hot-glue gun; and geometric shapes cut from various colors of railroad board or matte board

You can often get matte board scraps from framing shops or fine arts supply stores at minimal cost or for free! Many times, all you have to do is ask.

1. Place the shapes on the table within reach of the clients.
2. Spend some time reviewing shapes. Ask each individual to hold the shape. Can they tell you what color it is? Can they think of something else that is that color or shape? If that client cannot answer, ask for help from the rest of the group.
3. Place several pieces of different sizes, shapes, and colors directly in front of the client.
4. Using one-step directives, ask them to each pick a shape, identify its color and shape, and place it on the black surface.

5. Assist with applying glue, or tack the shapes on with hot glue. NOTE: Always keep the hot glue away from participants!

6. Continue taking turns to place shapes on the board until the surface is well covered. Black board works best for the background color because it makes applied shapes and colors easier to see for those whose vision is limited.

This technique can also be done with black poster board and colored construction paper, but you lose the tactile benefits that handling weightier items brings. The finished product is aesthetically pleasing and should not result in the dreaded "that's for little children" comments you may get from staff and other clients. The displayed product is further useful to other staff when interacting with those clients by providing them the opportunity to further reinforce the basic knowledge of color and shapes at any time.

I've Been Framed!: High- to Medium-Level Cognitive Functioning

Every piece of fine painting we have ever seen has a frame around it. Some incorporate very grandiose, ornate carvings covered in gold, while others can be very plain unpainted wood or metal. When done properly, the frame will reflect the feeling and content of the artwork it surrounds. If we consider ourselves as works of art (as we should!), what kind of frame would surround us? This is the question I posed to a high- to medium-level cognitive functioning group of geriatric and rehab clients, and the results were all that I had hoped for. The frames were reflective of the clients themselves and enhanced the total creation of who they are. Here is where we started.

Materials needed: various sizes and colors of cut matte board frames (some very large, 22″ × 24″, and some no smaller than 11″ × 14″) with margins of 3″ or greater (to provide enough work surface for each individual); scissors; acrylic paints; white glue; glitter; feathers; beads; buttons; ribbon; lace; leather; burlap; patterned paper (such as wallpaper samples); cotton; brushes; water containers; table coverings; and a large square mirror and/or Polaroid camera

1. Discuss the theory of viewing ourselves as artwork and the use of frames, as described above.
2. Ask the clients to create a frame that will enhance or further develop themselves as fine art.
3. Ask them to choose a base frame from the matte frames provided.
4. Lay out the collage materials described above. Ask clients to choose any that they want to use in the creation of their frames. Assist with glue, etc., as necessary.
5. Allow 20 minutes working time.
6. When clients are finished, ask each participant to share their frame with the group. Why did they use certain materials? What does the frame say about themselves as artwork?
7. Taking turns now, ask each person to hold the frame up to their faces/body. Does the frame fit our perceptions of the person?
8. Hold the mirror up to each person so they can see their "fine art framed." Take a Polaroid if you choose.

In my group, the clients really enjoyed seeing themselves in "portrait form" behind their frame, and the looks on their faces were indescribable. You may see some of that forgotten self-pride shine through as you allow the individual to assign him or herself some worth and value as human art. Some of the clients initiated trying on others' frames to see if they suited them; inevitably they didn't quite fit, which led to a discussion about individuality and personality differences. Everyone was encouraged to take their frame home if they chose.

Box Sculpture: Medium- to High-Level Cognitive Functioning

This technique calls for some advance preparation. You will need to spray-paint a variety of different shaped and sized boxes solid colors such as red, black, gold, yellow, green, etc.

Materials needed: boxes prepared as described above (plan for a minimum of three per client); hot glue; liquid glue; miscellaneous geometric and organic shapes cut from colored poster board or matte board scraps; feathers; and miscellaneous collage materials such as feathers, sequins, fur scraps, or sticks

1. Tell clients they are going to create a three-dimensional image of themselves using a box or boxes to create it. The image does not need to look like a body; it should just be a representation of themselves in form and feeling.
2. Distribute boxes, allowing clients to choose up to three of any shape, size, or color combination.
3. Ask them to lay out or stack the boxes in the general shape they'd like to begin with.
4. Hot-glue the boxes in place.
5. Distribute miscellaneous collage materials and glue sticks.
6. Assist in adding embellishments to the sculpture if necessary. Make holes in the boxes with the sharp end of a compass or other tool, and stick feathers into the boxes, if desired.
7. After the clients have finished, ask to view their representations. How are they like their 3-D creations? Why did they choose the boxes they did? Does the size and total creation "fit" the person?

One of the clients in my group had recently begun to have paranoid delusions that people were trying to kill her. Interestingly enough, she chose a box with a removable lid, as well as a much smaller black box. She chose to enclose the black box between the lid and the bottom of the other, as if sheltering it from its surroundings. She then proceeded to enclose the center even further with strips of paper so that the internal box was completely protected from the outside. Although this client couldn't verbalize her feelings of fear to the group, her sculpture revealed her new perceived need for protection.

Chapter 6

Miscellaneous Techniques

A WORD ABOUT MISCELLANEOUS TECHNIQUES

This section encompasses a wide variety of drawing, painting, stencil, and organic-art processes designed to offer clients many opportunities to express themselves using a number of different, imaginative, and enjoyable themes and plans. Some of the processes, like the ones found under the subheading of "Nature Objects," will require you to scavenge a bit, but will allow your clients contact with natural and organic "art media."

The "Stencils" section requires the use of a light source, the most effective of which is an overhead projector, and requires a good deal of assistance from the therapist, depending upon the abilities of the clients.

Although many of these plans give options for the use of several different mediums, you may want to limit the choices if your clients have difficulty making decisions, or if you feel too many choices may overstimulate them. Your professional judgment should always be used to determine if specific processes are right for the population you work with.

MARKERS, CRAYONS, AND PAINTS

Roadways: Medium- to High-Level Cognitive Functioning

This is a type of timeline/life review activity with many variables. Clients are asked to think about their journeys through life as road trips. This group can be simplified for more hesitant artists by offering a variety of predrawn "roads" (see next page), or you can offer full artistic license and allow them to complete their roads independently.

Materials needed: drawing paper (one per client or have several sheets per client available with road possibilities to choose from); markers; crayons; and/or craypas

1. Discuss the road of life with your clients. What does that phrase mean to them? Ask them to consider their personal roads and their journeys upon them. What kind of roads would they be? Gravel? Dirt? An expressway? How would they have travelled on these roads? By car? On foot? On horseback? Which direction are they going? How fast? Ask them to consider these questions and to create their roads.

   If you predict your group members will have difficulty beginning, offer them a predrawn alternative. Offering them a choice among many possible roads should not be considered intrusive, but just helpful in getting the clients started; the rest of the decisions will be their own.

2. Remind them to consider all the aspects mentioned above, as well as environment surrounding the roads.

3. Allow 20 minutes or so for clients to complete their roads.

4. When they have finished, ask about aspects of their work. How fast were they going? Can you guess by the mode of transportation? Were their roads going uphill or downhill? What was the terrain surrounding the roads like? Are they traveling alone? Are people's roads similar to one another, or are each unique? Would they change anything? Is there a toll? End the group by discussing roadways. Can the road change?

The road turns every day to delight and inspire us, and to challenge and help us to understand that whatever road we travel, we do not travel alone and we are more the wiser at the end of the journey. Below are some example roadways you can supply to help get your clients started. (See Illustration 6.1.)

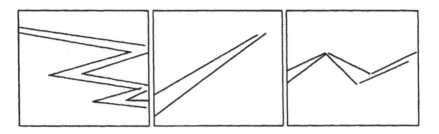

Illustration 6.1. Roadway Samples

Images of Life, Pieces of the Puzzle: Medium- to High-Level Cognitive Functioning

This is a good process to experience when developing a new group. It allows individuals the opportunity to express their thoughts independently and see how other's ideas often reflect their own.

Materials needed: poster board precut into workable puzzle pieces (allow one piece per participant); acrylic paint; markers or crayons; brushes; and table coverings

Create a puzzle by cutting a sheet of poster board into irregular shapes with common borders. For larger groups or larger pieces, tape poster board together into a large sheet and cut it into pieces.

1. Before the group activity begins, set the materials and one piece of the puzzle per person (not in order) on the table.
2. Initiate a discussion reflecting on all the different components there are in life; that is, discuss all the different aspects we experience daily and how these aspects affect us. Some examples may be youth, creativity, sound, ability to grow, and ability to express thoughts.

3. Ask clients to think about what aspects of life mean the most to them or affect them the most.
4. Working with the poster board provided, ask them to create an image that would reflect their feelings.
5. When everyone has finished, ask each client to discuss his or her image with the group and to explain its importance to them. When the client has finished the discussion ask him or her to put the piece of art on the table.
6. Repeat this with the remaining members of the group.
7. When all of the pieces are on the table, ask the group members if they can fit the pieces together. Assist them if necessary.
8. Discuss the result. You may find that the participants will recognize aspects of other's images and thoughts that reflect their own, and how all of the issues and images affect all of us at one time or another–how all of the pieces of life, good and bad, are needed to create the whole as we know it. You may also find that some images don't "go" with the others (visually), but they are still an important part of the whole, and thereby necessary. Ask clients how this relates to our existence.
9. Close the group with the shared knowledge that although everyone is an individual, we all share experiences, both the painful and joyful kinds, and that these help create our strength and wisdom.

Life Series: Medium- to High-Level Cognitive Functioning

This group focuses on organized thinking and looks at three-step processes. It allows participants to concretely deal with life issues and the "passing of time." During the processing stage of this group, feelings regarding death and the end of life may arise, so be sure the group is cohesive and supportive enough to deal with these issues.

Materials needed: 18" × 24" sheets of watercolor paper (one sheet per client) divided into three equal sections with black permanent marker; crayons; markers; watercolor or acrylic paints; water containers; brushes; table coverings; and music playing in background

1. Provide each participant with a piece of the divided water-color paper.
2. Discuss how, in life, many things we experience go through a series of changes or development. Brainstorm ideas with the group to assist them in better understanding the concept. Some ideas may be seasons changing, flowers growing, or humans aging.
3. Discuss ways to symbolize changes we go through and/or changes they feel are significant to them.
4. Instruct them to use the spaces provided on their paper to express a series of changes in any way they like: through color or line, symbolically, or realistically.
5. Play music in the background and allow them to work quietly.
6. When all clients are finished, discuss the relevance of their artwork and how the series relates to them.

You may find pictures of time passing; e.g., a tree growing, flowers blooming and then dying, buildings being constructed or torn down. (See Photo 6.1.) Discuss with the group the concept of birth, growth, death, and rebirth. Many groups connect this to biblical teachings, but it relates in the everyday world also, such as the passing of the seasons.

Close the group with a discussion on the eternal nature of life and legacy. The group may touch on feelings regarding their own demise, so be sensitive and supportive. Focus on the positive changes there are in life and the joy of seeing things grow.

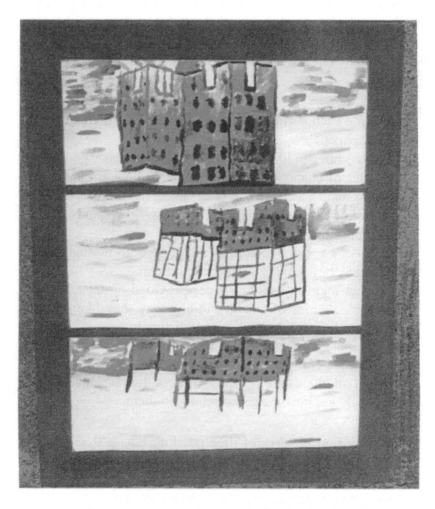

Photo 6.1. Life Series. Shows the Demise of a Building, Significantly Reflecting the Multiple Amputations this Diabetic Client was Experiencing (Client Started at Bottom)

Doorways to Imagination: Medium- to High-Level Cognitive Functioning

This process deals mostly with individual identity and self-expression of the private places we escape to in our imagination. It should only be done with cohesive groups that know each other well. It can be done in a two-session format.

Materials needed: large sheets of paper or poster board; pencils; markers; crayons; scissors; tape; rulers; compasses; and examples of different kinds of doorways (look in children's books and art history books for a variety of samples)

1. Have materials on the tables when clients arrive.
2. Lead clients through some relaxation exercises, focusing on breathing and becoming calm. Play soft, neutral music in the background. (New-age music works well here, as it does not always suggest any particular mood).
3. Instruct the clients to close their eyes and imagine a doorway or door that leads to a special place where only they can go. This doorway is different from any doorway they've ever seen. It belongs to them.
4. Ask them to think about the color of the doorway or door. How does it open? What kind of handle or knob does it have? Can you see through it? Is it locked? Is it ornate or simple? Scary or inviting?
5. Ask them to use the provided materials to create that doorway.
6. When the clients are finished, ask them questions about their doorways, such as the ones mentioned in step 4. Ask them if they are the only ones who can enter. Is the door heavy and difficult to open? Does it imply what may lay beyond it?
7. At the next session, hand out pieces of paper.

8. Ask the clients to think back to their doorways and to the secret places they lead to. Allow them to express that environment on the second piece of paper.
9. When done, ask each client to discuss his or her secret place. Is he or she willing to let others in? Is it a place he or she would go to often? What does it provide that he or she doesn't have or experience in this world?
10. Offer the opportunity to make an opening in the doorways (with the scissors) so that each person's place is more accessible.

If the group allows you to display their work, attach the doorway over the secret place so that anyone who wants to look inside will have to go through the clients' personal doors.

End the session by discussing the new awareness of our secret retreats and mention that although we cannot live there, it will always exist for us as a quiet and comforting place.

Additional Possibilities

This process can also be done as a multimedia collage, incorporating fabric and textures, or even done in a realistic-size mural if your clients are ambulatory or have good range of motion.

Cave Painting: Medium- to High-Level Cognitive Functioning

This process centers around a discussion of the use of symbols in drawings to describe an event or to tell a story. This was a significant method of communication used by prehistoric cavemen, and is a wonderful way for us today to get a glimpse of what their lives were like. Go to the library and look for photographic essays of some of the more famous cave painting areas and have these pictures available to show clients that although primitively done, the paintings amaze and fascinate the viewer.

To get the clients in the mood to become cavemen themselves, I provided fake furs to drape around their shoulders. Our discussion began with general caveman knowledge. What did they wear? (Provide fur scraps.) What did they eat and use for tools? (I made some large bones out of poster board.) What did they paint? (They painted things they saw every day, such as animals.) Then move into the art experience.

Materials needed: large sheet of brown butcher paper (crumpled to give it a cave-wall texture); colored chalks (reds, browns, and blacks); fur scraps; bones; and a Polaroid camera, if possible

1. Lay paper out on a long table.
2. Provide each client with colored chalks.
3. Begin your discussion of cavemen, by showing pictures of cave paintings and discussing lifestyle as described above. Distribute fur and bones and ask each member to think of him or herself as a prehistoric man/woman. Chose names, e.g., "Larry the mammoth hunter of the fourth-floor clan."
4. Next, ask them to tell a story using symbols such as those the cavemen might have used. Ask them to draw something that they may see everyday, or to draw out a situation so that the viewer might learn what the "modern" cave painters' lives are like.
5. Allow the group 20 minutes to work. Remind them that they are cavemen now and cannot talk with words, though grunting is allowed!
6. When the clients are finished, address each one by his or her cave name and ask the other members of the clan if they can guess what the story of the other's painting might be. Even though they are cave painters, the situations they will be drawing will be contemporary. They are, after all, modern cavemen!
7. When completely through, take a Polaroid picture of these cavemen before they go back to the real world. Display it

along with their cave wall if desired, or allow them to keep it as a reminder of their participation.

Gift Boxes: Medium- to High-Level Cognitive Functioning

The giving of a gift, for whatever reason, provides us with an opportunity to consider the people we care for and about. Gift-giving can provide an opportunity to express to your friends and family your thoughts about them and why your relationship exists.

Relationships that develop during hospitalization or long-term care placement are equally important to your clients. Many groups meet only once a week, and sometimes the personal relationships between these participants ends there; however, the fact remains that these people know each other very well. If your group changes rapidly, you can see that the necessity to "open up" to acquaintances is sometimes part of the art therapy process, thereby making people "instant" friends in the sense that they, too, know each other well.

This process helps us take a look at the tradition of giving in the context of a group of friendly strangers. It helps solidify relationships in the group, and acknowledges the desire to share with others.

Materials needed: heavyweight watercolor paper, cut into boxes (see instructions below) or flattened white boxes; Craypas; crayons; markers; and clear adhesive tape

1. Prepare box shapes ahead of group time, keep flat, but pre-cut and folded. To do this, take a square piece of paper (size is your option) and fold four times lengthwise and width-wise. Cut the corners as shown in Illustration 6.2.
2. Write the participants' names on slips of paper and have group members choose names. (If your group members do not all have positive feelings toward each other, take the liberty of hand-selecting names to exchange.)

3. Ask them to think about the person whose name they have chosen, and to create, as a gift, a positive collage of words and images that represents that other person. They may also add words or images of things that they may want to give that person if they could. Emphasize that these are not material things, but rather feelings or thoughts.

4. Allow clients to work for approximately 20 minutes.

5. As they finish, fold their paper into box shapes and tape them together. You can ask the creator if he or she would like to give the gift with the imagery on the outside or on the inside. Do they want everyone to see their feelings? Do they think the person for whom they made this gift would like others to see it?

6. When all participants are through, ask them to present their gift boxes to the people. Ask them to read some of the words or explain some of the imagery created, if they feel comfortable.

7. You may then give each person a little "treat" to put inside the box as a personal thank you for their participation, as I did.

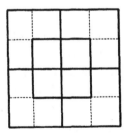

Illustration 6.2. Gift Box Pattern

This inevitably leads to a lot of positive thoughts between the group members, and raises individuals' self-esteem by hearing themselves talked about by others in such a positive manner.

Each participant then has a nice reminder of those positive strokes in the shape of an open box. What better gift to give?

Afraid of the Dark?: Medium- to High-Level Cognitive Functioning

The use of glow-in-the-dark paints makes this a fun group activity that surprises your clients and allows them to laugh during the process of creativity. A room with few or no windows is needed for this, as you want a dark enough environment to be able to make the most of the glow paints. CAUTION: Know your clients well before doing this, as some individuals may become uncomfortable with being put in the dark for even a few minutes. If you suspect your clients would be uncomfortable, warn them ahead of time and focus on the safety of the group. This process is not intended for use with truly troubled individuals who may have had good reason to fear the dark.

Materials needed: glow-in-the-dark acrylic paints or fabric paints; black construction paper or poster board; white pencils; pastel chalks; paintbrushes; and water containers

1. Have black paper, white pencils, and pastel chalks out on the tables as clients come in.
2. Begin a discussion of "the dark." What do we associate with darkness? Childhood fears? Monsters under the bed? Mysterious things? Good spirits? Romance?
3. Using the materials provided, ask the clients to create the things that they associate with "being part of the dark."
4. Bring out the glow-in-the-dark materials. Ask clients to highlight their images with the paints provided. (Don't tell them that they will glow!)
5. When all are done, discuss the images. Do we share the same ideas of the dark?

6. Now, for fun, turn off lights in the room. Their images should appear to float and "glow in the dark." Ask the clients to hold their pictures in front of them so that the others may enjoy the images also.
7. Next, turn the lights back on and discuss the fact that the images did not really change when going from light to dark. Is it just our perception of them that changed? Why?

Close the group by letting clients know that the dark doesn't have to be frightening if you are with people you trust.

The First Line: High- to Medium-Level Cognitive Functioning

Nothing is as frightening to an artist or artist-to-be as a blank piece of paper. Too many times, the first mark they make is like life and death—it could be the beginning of something wonderful, or the beginning of a torturous event that they then have to overcome. I had a design teacher once tell me that to erase a line is like killing a living thing. Even a line on a piece of paper has some value as a building block. Good or bad, that line has a purpose.

The following treatment plan takes away that "first-line fright" because you provide that line for your client. Sometimes having a line already made for you can be more of a challenge than beginning from scratch by yourself. This process challenges abstract thinking skills and imagination, and provides both structure and freedom to aid creation. It can be done with both high-level cognitive functioning clients as well as medium-level clients, depending upon the amount of form and structure you provide with your first line.

Materials needed: watercolor paper 8″ × 10″ or 11″ × 14″ (one piece per participant); black waterproof markers (such as "Sharpies"); watercolor paints; water containers; brushes; and table coverings

1. Before the group activity begins, prepare one sheet of watercolor paper for each client. On each sheet, use a marker to initiate the "first line." (See Illustration 6.3 for some of the lines I used.)

2. When the clients arrive, tell them you are going to challenge their imagination! Pass out the prepared paper. If you know your clients well, you should choose lines that may match their ability to think complexly. For example, I know Jane has a difficult time with complex abstract thinking so I may draw example E on her paper because it is an easily recognizable form—it could be a fence, railroad tracks, etc.

3. Instruct the clients to use the markers to change or enlarge the linear design already present if they wish, and to use the watercolors directly over the drawing to finish off the image and to give it background or a "setting."

4. Play soft music in the background and allow 20 minutes or so to work.

5. If someone is having problems getting started, make the linear design more substantial, more specific to an image, or ask the rest of the group for ideas.

6. When the clients are finished, ask each individual to share his or her image with the rest of the group. Ask the clients if they had difficulty starting, or if they immediately got an idea from the lines. Allow the other group members to share what they would have done if they had gotten those "first lines."

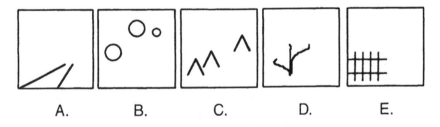

Illustration 6.3. First Lines

Even though this group starts out with prepared lines on paper, the artist inevitably puts his or her own personality and issues onto the image. In my group, Jane created a fence and a wild-flower garden from example E, while another client saw those lines as being jail-cell bars. Jane often talks about her beautiful garden at her home and the joy she had there. The other client makes it well known that her "institutionalization" is very restrictive to her and she often feels like she is in jail.

Other possibilities exist for line examples, including the following: A: A road leading . . . ?; B: Moons over a distant planet; C: Mountains or teepees; D: A flower stem; and E: A fence, rail-road tracks, or jail cell.

Ask your co-workers to create first lines for you if you need some ideas, or if appropriate, ask the clients to create simple lines and pass their papers to another participant for the project. I hesitate in doing this myself because, without knowing what the lines will be used for, your clients may create much too complex line designs and cause someone else great frustration! Hopefully, the lines you provide will stimulate imagination and creativity in your clients and in yourself.

STENCILS

Spray Paint Stencil Mural: Medium- to High-Level Cognitive Functioning

Although this process is time-consuming and requires much assistance from the therapist, the results are truly impressive and offer the clients a very rounded representation of themselves and the individuals in their group.

A stencil is created by casting a client's shadow against a wall to which paper is attached, and tracing around the shadow. In this activity, two stencils are created of each client; one will be a silhouette, the other will reflect something about the client, his or her interests, and what's important to him or her.

Materials needed: a light source; lightweight white paper; masking tape; pencils; spray paints; and scissors

1. Tell the clients that they are going to do a true portrait of themselves as members of the group. It will be a group collage when completed.
2. Take turns casting silhouettes and carefully trace the clients' shadows in detail. Cut the silhouettes out from the paper.
3. Next, ask them to identify something about themselves and to create a symbol for that interest. For example, Joe likes music so he chose music notes to represent himself. Ask clients to draw these on paper and cut them out, creating a stencil.
4. Now, in a well-ventilated area, lay the background paper (a large white sheet of paper, preferably in one sheet from a roll) on the ground and one-by-one, lay the silhouettes on the paper.
5. Ask each client what color he or she would like the silhouette to be highlighted in, and spray the color around the portrait until a clear outline is created.
6. Continue with the rest of the group.
7. Next, lay the interest stencil over each portrait and spray lightly with a different color of their choice. Continue with the entire group.
8. Next, overlap one client's portrait over another's and lightly spray with an alternate color until the silhouette is seen faintly. Continue with the rest of the group.

NOTE: It is important to do this in a well-ventilated area, as you will be spraying the paint several times. I did this process in a large room with the clients seated around the base paper in a circle while I sprayed their chosen colors for them. If your clients are more able, do this process outside and let them spray the paint. Unfortunately, there is no other way to get this particular effect other than to use spray paint. Sponging the different colors onto the paper loses the airbrush quality and does not define the portraits as well.

When complete, ask the clients what their thoughts are about the process. How does it reflect the entity of the group? Display the mural along with an explanation of the process.

Shadow Portraits: Medium- to High-Level Cognitive Functioning

This process encourages body awareness and movement, while considering personal issues. It places the artist in the role of "art" itself, and provides opportunities to share hidden and unfamiliar parts of ourselves with others. It helps reveal our "dark side" in a safe and supportive environment.

Materials needed: large sheets of plain, somewhat thin, white paper (approximately 36″ × 36″); large sheets of black paper (one color of each for each person in the group); a large overhead projector or light source; a blank wall where paper can be hung; white pencil; regular pencils; and several pairs of scissors

1. Begin the group activity with participants in a circle, with the light source and wall area cleared for access. Begin a discussion of personalities and their positive and negative sides (e.g., "I have a great sense of humor, but I also have a bad temper"). Explore how each one of us has these alternate sides and how some people only see our good sides, and some people only see our bad sides. Have each client in the group think about their "light and dark sides."
2. Next, discuss how body language can imply different moods and feelings. For example, a fist might signal anger, while open arms may signal affection.

3. Ask each client to come to the blank wall (assist them if necessary).

4. Tape the large black sheet of paper to the wall. Seat the participant very close to it, either facing the wall or in profile.

5. Ask them to show you, through body language, what they may perceive as their "dark side." Remember, the "dark side" does not have to be a negative aspect, just one that perhaps others don't see frequently or that we don't access much. It could be shyness, loneliness, fear, pensiveness, religious practices, etc.

6. Shine the light toward them to cast a shadow onto the paper.

7. Trace the silhouette with the white pencil. Make sure to take the time to get small details, like the curls in the hair, or even any adaptive equipment they may use.

8. Now turn them another way, either facing the wall or in profile.

9. Tape the white sheet in place behind them.

10. Ask them to portray an aspect of their "lighter side" through body positioning.

11. Trace the silhouette.

12. Repeat the process with all participants.

13. Assist them in carefully cutting out these silhouettes.

14. Superimpose the white silhouette over the dark one, possibly dropping the top one down and over somewhat until you can see detail from both silhouettes. You should also be able to see some of the black silhouette through the white paper. Tape them together and display.

When all silhouettes are assembled, discuss the necessity of both sides of our personality, by explaining that together they make us who we are.

Participants in the group that I did this process with were very proud of the finished product, even though it may have been revealing to others, because they recognized their abilities to become "art," not just "creators" of it. This process is also enlightening when used with a "fantasy" theme, such as how you see yourself or how you'd wish to be seen.

NATURE OBJECTS

Talisman: Medium- to High-Level Cognitive Functioning

The definition of a "talisman" is a symbol or charm, a protecting object or symbol of protection. Talismans have been a form of comfort and focus of belief for many cultures through the ages. Talismans have traditionally been created as a visual connection to what individuals see as a guiding force in their lives. An example of a type of talisman could be the animal symbols many tribal cultures have taken on, exhibiting their belief that the power and personality of the animal somehow is a directing force within themselves. Another example could be the present-day crucifix symbol that many wear as a symbol of their religious beliefs.

This process focuses on the historical meaning and usefulness of the talisman. Begin a discussion on the background of the word, in reference to the way that individuals may assign themselves a connection with animal, nature, or spirit.

Materials needed: leather scraps cut in manageable pieces; natural feathers; artificial eagle feathers; fabrics; yarns and threads; wire; small pieces of cardboard; hot-glue gun; and permanent markers

1. Begin the discussion of talismans and their historical significance. Relate the symbol of the talisman with that of a personal connection with an animal spirit or the spirit of something in nature; e.g., lightening, a waterfall, an eagle, a mouse, a tornado, etc.

2. Ask each participant to consider a relationship between him or herself and either a force of nature, a source of life, or anything else they feel could relate to part of their personalities. Give some examples. For example, "I am shy, like a deer; I am unpredictable, like a storm." You could also have them select a talisman of a complementary nature; e.g., "I am weak, therefore I need the protection of the bear."

3. Using the materials provided, ask the clients to create a symbol of the spirit they have chosen. They can use the cardboard or the leather as a base for this. Anything is possible here; the process could be as simple as drawing symbols on the leather, or as complex as creating a multi-media symbol.

4. Assist as necessary with the gluing of materials. NOTE: The reason hot glue is used here is because it adheres immediately and permanently to all surfaces; use with caution and discretion.

5. When each person is finished, ask him or her to share the symbol, the reason for choosing it, and how he or she felt solidifying the experience with the collage. If they chose a complementary symbol, ask them to consider accepting the "spirit" of that choice and allowing it to make them feel stronger.

Sometimes showing pictures of other traditional talismans helps get the clients started. These can be found in any local library or art history book. Consider playing "nature" or environmental tapes during this activity. This creates a quiet, respectful feeling for the participants.

Adaptations

This process can also be done with clay, in the tradition of "fetishes."

Rock Solid: Medium- to High-Level Cognitive Functioning

There is something comforting and simply beautiful in utilizing the wealth of nature to inspire self-reflection and self-acceptance. This group incorporates large natural rock formations to assist in this back-to-nature art experience. Playing environmental tapes for this process also makes it more cohesive and helps to create the right mood for the group. NOTE: This process is not suggested for use with violence-risk individuals, as the rocks suggested would be large and heavy.

Materials needed: large (hand-size and slightly larger) rocks (enough for all members of the group); feathers; textured fine yarns; "Slickers"; and 3-D paints

1. You can find rocks in parks and at the beach. Try to find rocks with interesting lines, crevices, and colors. Wash and dry the rocks thoroughly before the group activity.
2. Set the rocks on a table. Allow clients to select a rock that appeals to them.
3. When everyone has selected a rock, ask them to examine the rocks closely, feel the weight of them, and notice the contours and crevices.
4. Next, ask each person to describe his or her rock to the group, again showing others the individual markings that make it different from other rocks.
5. Discuss the following questions: How old do you think the rock might be? Where might it have come from? What might it have experienced during its "lifetime?" If it could talk, what might it say? If it could see, what might it have seen? What might have caused its cracks, holes, crevices, dents, and other characteristics?
6. Now that the clients have gotten to know their individual rocks, with all of their faults and flaws, allow the partici-

pants to "dress them up" a little by wrapping the rocks with yarns, tying on feathers, or adding color with paints. Encourage them not to cover the whole rock over, so that you will still be able to identify it. Clients may need help with beginning the yarn around the rock. Feathers can easily be attached by running the quill pin under the yarns. Depending on the physical capabilities of your group, you might plan on having some "extra hands" in the form of volunteers to help with the yarn-tying, as two hands are needed to support and wind the yarn around the rock.

7. Next, have each client show his or her *new* rock. Ask how he or she feels about the changes. Discuss how the rock still maintains its character despite the additions.

8. Ask each individual how he or she could relate him or herself to the rock. Lead the client into a discussion if necessary by asking questions such as, "Your rock has some scars running over it as if it has been scratched through the years. Do you feel you have gained any scratches over the years?" or "Your rock has seen changes in its environment; how has your environment changed?"

9. End the group by discussing how, despite all the changes and ages the rocks have been through, they are still solid, and that the cracks only make them more interesting and strong.

Branching Out: Medium- to High-Level Cognitive Functioning; Low with Adaptations

Trees, in all their varied forms, are universally experienced and have in most cases provided fond memories of protection, security, and life in the "outside world" to the clients we work with. Trees can also be related to our *own* feelings of strength or weakness, age and beauty, when used in an art therapy process.

Knowing this, I embarked on an interesting journey of both sculpture-making and self-reflection with my geriatric residential-care clients.

Materials needed: four large, straight tree branches (approximately 4' to 5' long); a selection of large tree branches (at least as many as there are members in your group, plus another five for greater selection) with interesting features such as peeling bark, bends, breaks, etc.; raffia (a natural fiber string); hot-glue gun; and scissors

Before the group activity begins, take the four straight branches and tie them together at the corners with raffia to create a rough frame. Hot-glue the joints for extra stability. Put aside. Lay the rest of your branches on the table that you will seat your clients around.

1. Begin the group by discussing peoples' feelings about trees. What are some things we associate with trees? Possible answers would be stability, shelter, growth, a provider, and protection.
2. Ask the clients to look through the branches provided and pick out one that interests them and whose structure appeals to them. Ask them to look closely at their branches, from the point-of-view of an artist, and describe them to the rest of the group. Ask them to consider the following: limb shape—is it flexible or brittle? Is it heavy, weathered, ragged, or broken? What kinds of things might this branch have experienced to make it look that way?
3. Have clients take turns describing their branches. In my experience, clients will describe the branch as they might describe themselves (e.g., "This tree started out strong, then nature had an effect on it and changed its course forever . . . yet it is still strong and sturdy"). As they describe their tree,

ask them if any of what they say relates to them. Do they still feel strong and flexible even though they are "weathered"?
4. As each person speaks, have him or her lay his or her branch on the frame. You can then tie it on with raffia and later secure it with hot glue.
5. After everyone has placed the branches on the frame, ask if the branches look stronger with the others to support them. Do all the individual characteristics complement each other to form the sculpture?

My results were positive. As a group, the clients agreed that each branch, like each person, is different and has its own special characteristics. Yet branches, like people, are still able to come together, support each other, and continue to grow.

Later, I hung the piece of artwork with an explanation of the process and some quotes from the group. Displaying this piece in lower-level client areas provides great reality orientation to seasons and can become part of sensory stimulation groups. It is also useful to other therapists working in your facility as a point of interest during walks or rehabilitation training. Of course, consider loose bark and roughness of wood before displaying in areas where your clients may need more supervision.

Adaptations

This process can also be used, on a smaller scale, with lower-level functioning clients. Choose smaller branches to use as a frame and concentrate on sensory stimulation and one-step directive completion (e.g., Pick up a stick; How does it feel? Is it heavy or light? What color is it? Is it smooth or rough? Place it on the frame).

Although this is not "traditional" art, both clients and staff are drawn to it because of its organic look and the deeply felt connection to nature and to each other.

STRING

Stringing Along: High-Level Cognitive Functioning

This is an excellent decision-making and gross motor-skills process. It does, however, require a certain amount of range of motion and the use of two hands. Adaptive equipment is available to clamp the frames in an upright and stationary position so that the client can simply wrap threads around a motionless frame, or you can plan ahead to have students or volunteers available who can hold and rotate frames for your clients, if necessary.

Materials needed: flat or squared-off frames similar to those used for stretching canvas or those used for picture frames; a variety of fine-quality weaving yarn with different textures and colors in smaller diameters (do not use thick acrylic yarn, as it makes the finished product look childish); masking tape; scissors; and table clamps (if needed)

1. Have yarn available on each table. If necessary, cut into two-yard lengths for easier handling by clients.
2. Ask clients to choose a frame. Provide frames in a variety of colors. (Spray paint the frames ahead of time in colors such as black, red, and dark blue.)
3. Ask clients to choose yarn that complements the frame they have selected. Ask them to take notice of the different textures available and to carefully choose two or three types.
4. Tape one end of each piece of yarn to the back of the clients' frames. Ask clients to wrap the yarn around their frames to create a webbing.
5. Tape the other end of each piece of string to the back of each frame.
6. Begin the next piece of yarn at a different point on the frame. Have clients repeat with all three types of yarn, crisscrossing the previous yarn as they go.

7. When all clients are finished, ask them to take a look at their finished products. Can they title them? What do they remind them of?

You may get a variety of line designs from your clients, ranging from straight–linear without crossing each thread–to a chaotic webbing of colors and textures. Individual personalities really come through here, and the titles can often be surprisingly revealing for such a limited process!

Other ways of doing this process are to make geometric frames out of dowels, or to wrap threads around precut matte boards. Using metallic threads minimally also can create great results and variety. (See Photo 6.2.)

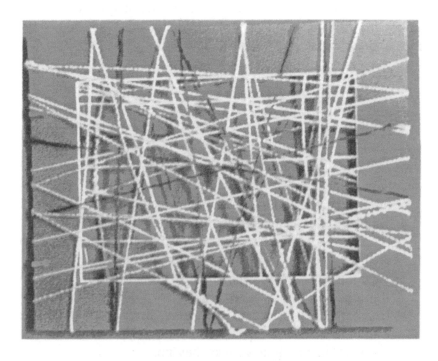

Photo 6.2. Stringing Along

OTHER TECHNIQUES

Shout It Out: Medium- to High-Level Cognitive Functioning

Most of us suppress our feelings at one time or another. Is it because it is socially acceptable for us to sit quietly in our rage or in our joy? We are not to brag, to yell, to dance in the streets. Art is much less restrictive than that, and as a therapist, you should never forget that you can CHANGE THE RULES.

In a safe place, we can set our emotions free, and, if appropriate for your clients, you can give them a chance to identify suppressed feelings and literally shout them out.

This group is asked to discuss shouting. Why do people shout? Because of joy, good news, anger, or frustration? Can it be both positive and negative? How does it feel? When was the last time you really shouted? Are you uncomfortable with shouting? What does shouting do? (It causes attention to be drawn to the shout-ee.) Your group will then create megaphones.

Materials needed: construction paper of various sizes and colors; markers; crayons; 3-D paints; and clear tape

Use the construction paper to create a template of various sizes to either be traced and cut by you or by your clients, depending on their abilities. See Illustration 6.4 for template; enlarge it to the desired size.

1. Begin the discussion as explained above.
2. Discuss megaphones. What are they used for? (They are used to make your voice louder.) Ask them to think of something that they would like to shout. It can be anything–a shout of joy, of frustration–whatever they want. Now ask clients to create megaphones that will reflect the words they might

shout through it. How loud do they want to shout? This will determine the size of the megaphone. What kind of feelings will they express? This will determine the color and the images they will choose to decorate their megaphones.

3. Allow them to choose their paper. You might need to assist with tracing. They can also choose from precut megaphones you may have prepared ahead of time. If you do this, make sure you have plenty of megaphones in various sizes and colors.
4. Pass out markers and paints.
5. Allow the clients 20 minutes to work.
6. When everyone is finished, shape and tape the megaphones together.
7. Next, ask them if they feel comfortable enough to take advantage of their megaphones and shout!
8. If clients are hesitant, show them how to use their megaphones! It's not easy, is it? But if it's done in a safe place, among friends and with laughter, it can be really liberating.

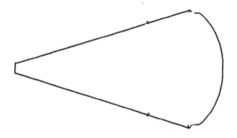

Illustration 6.4. Megaphone Pattern

Reach Out and Touch Us: Medium- to High-Level Cognitive Functioning

This process combines cast-shadow silhouettes and tactile fabric materials to achieve a unique self-portrait that just begs to be touched.

Material needed: overhead light or slide projector light source; white poster board; miscellaneous fabrics and materials (such as lace, leather, felt, burlap, sandpaper, silk, and yarn); glue; and scissors

1. Discuss the creation of a self-portrait that not only looks like the artist, but also feels like him or her–not really what their skin feels like, but what their personality or individuality may feel like. Ask them questions such as: "What kind of person are you?" "Are you soft and cuddly?" "Are you rough?" "Are you lacy or more like leather?" Ask them to think about these things as you cast their shadows onto the poster board. Trace and assist clients with cutting the silhouettes out if necessary.

2. Once the silhouette is cut out, distribute all materials within reach and encourage clients to work with the fabrics that feel most like themselves. They may overlap pieces and combine many different types if they choose. Don't worry about trimming pieces to the silhouette. Just glue them on and then trim off the excess when the clients are done so that the silhouette is once again present.

3. When everyone is finished, ask each person to explain what made them choose particular materials. Are they more of one kind than another? Do the other members of the group see them the same way?

4. Have clients title their works. Ask for permission to display them. (See Photos 6.3 and 6.4.)

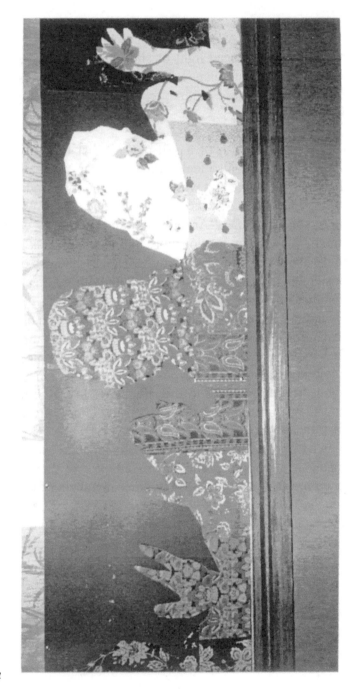

PHOTO 6.3. "Reach Out and Touch Us" Mural

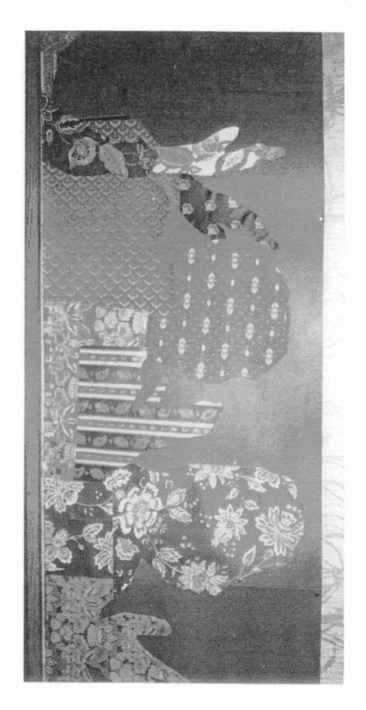

PHOTO 6.4. Details from "Reach Out and Touch Us" Mural

Appendix

Suggested Supplies

The following is a list of supplies needed to complete the treatment plans offered in this book, or those which every art therapist should have on hand. Suppliers and brands may be different than those mentioned here. However, most materials have many manufacturers. This list includes some brands that I have dealt with and use myself. All of these supplies are available at most large art supply stores.

(Starred items [*] can be adapted or are made in adaptive forms.)

PAPERS:

Lightweight student-grade watercolor paper

Heavyweight watercolor paper

Butcher-block paper on roll

Thin white paper on roll

Student-grade drawing paper

Regular-weight typing or xerox paper

Construction paper

Poster board

PAINTS/INKS:

Student-grade watercolor paints

"Prange"

Paints in tubes

Acrylic paints

"Luma" inks

FABRIC SUPPLIES/PAINTS:

Plain white cotton sheeting

"Slickers" paints in applicator bottles

"Tie-Dye Cords"

3-D fabric paint

Heat-sensitive and glow-in-the-dark fabric paints

ITEMS FROM DONATIONS:

Textured and patterned fabric samples, which can be obtained from upholstery stores

Discontinued matte board, which can be obtained from framing stores or art supply companies

CLAY:

White clay

Some no-fire clays, if available (terra-cotta "Ovencraft II" clay is nice if you don't intend to glaze the finished product)

MISCELLANEOUS:

Rubber gloves

Paper towels

Plastic table covers

Spray bottles for water

*Assortment of brushes

Colored pencils

*Markers

Wood dowels

Newspapers

*Scissors

Hot-glue gun

Prestretched and primed canvas

Large containers (such as cottage cheese containers) for holding water

Natural objects (shells, feathers, bark, etc.)

Adhesive tape

Plastic trays or palettes for paints

Index

Page numbers followed by the letter "p" indicate photos; those followed by the letter "i" indicate illustrations.

T - #0598 - 101024 - C0 - 212/152/7 - PB - 9780789001863 - Gloss Lamination